DOCTORS AS MANAGERS OF HEALTH TEAMS

ROMAN L. YANDA, M.D.

DOCTORS AS MANAGERS OF HEALTH TEAMS

**A Career Guide for
Hospital-Based Physicians**

A DIVISION OF AMERICAN MANAGEMENT ASSOCIATIONS

Library of Congress Cataloging in Publication Data

Yanda, Roman L
   Doctors as managers of health teams.

   Includes index.
   1. Hospitals--Medical staff. 2. Hospital care.
3. Health care teams. I. Title. [DNLM: 1. Hospital
administration--United States. 2. Physicians--United
States. WX155 Y21d]
RA972.Y36   610.69'52   76-54735
ISBN 0-8144-5432-1

© 1977 AMACOM

A division of American Management Associations, New York.
All rights reserved. Printed in the United States of America.

First Printing

PREFACE

THE NEED TO KNOW

*Some people continuously make the same mistake and
call it experience.*   Michael E. De Bakey, M.D.

The boom in health services, with its accompanying growth of
specialization, has greatly magnified the role of the hospital-based
physician. Effective management of specialty services has become
an urgent necessity too important to entrust to amateurs. Yet the
formal medical educational process is geared to the output of a professional type who is so inner-directed that adjusting to the team
role called for in the community may take years. A disruptive conflict between these two different perspectives of "reality" is avoided
only by the intrinsic adaptability and practicality of the doctors
who become leaders of men. But the price paid in wasted time and
motion and in increased friction is becoming too high for a cost-
conscious society.

Additionally, the once simple struggle for dominance between
medical staff and administration, which Lamb finds extending back
beyond 1875,[1] is now becoming increasingly complex and intense
with the major involvement of government and commercial interests under the swelling pressure of social, economic, and technological change. Without background information or a program guide,
the hospital-based physician can only respond willy-nilly to the
greatest pressures of the moment, and thus he is merely a pawn in
the struggle. When both population and pressure were smaller, the
neophyte had a reasonable chance of acquiring the necessary data

base during his long period of apprenticeship. But the "mass production" of doctors, the mounting flood of new information, and
the public's insistent demand for more specialists have gradually
pressured medical education into becoming even more of an ivory
tower than it used to be, to the exclusion of all other equally relevant human concerns.

Since my transit through, and graduation from, the system, I
have kept track of the major mistakes made in the area of hospital-
based practice, both my own and those of my peers. Spurred by
the definition of an expert as "one who has made all the mistakes,
and who knows it," I have, with the invaluable assistance of many
colleagues, assembled a compendium on this field. The purpose of
this book is to offer practical information and advice to the doctor
about to embark on a hospital-based career. Logically such subjects
should be part of the medical curriculum. To be effective leaders,
we must deliver the results required and desired by the consumer,
rather than just the "doing our own thing" that is so characteristic
of the haughty professional. There are others waiting on the
sidelines fully willing to exercise their guidance and control over
our technical talents should we fail to deliver the needed services
consistently.

This work is a continuation of a study in my own field of expertise[2] and would not have been possible without the willing assistance of many health professionals. It is impractical to list each
individual from whom I garnered facts, history, and perspective,
but there are three whose efforts deserve specific thanks: David
Moody for his incisive editorial work, Tai.K.Oh for the constructive help on management aspects, and Jane Beaulieu for cheerfully
retyping draft after draft.

Roman L. Yanda

CONTENTS

1

THE
LEADERSHIP
FUNCTION

THE MAGNITUDE OF THE DEMAND

Hospitals and hospital-based physicians have evolved dramatically over the centuries. The basic triumvirate at the beginning of the century was the pathologist, the anesthesiologist, and the radiologist. However, with the explosion in medical knowledge and technology since World War II there has been an exponential increase in the numbers and the types of specialized hospital-based physicians at even the community hospital level. This change has recently accelerated in the past decade until currently there are:

Pathology	Radiology
Anesthesiology	Cardiology
Emergency Room	Special Care
Services	Units (ICU/CCU)
Pediatric Unit	Gastroenterology/
Renal Dialysis/	Endoscopy
Nephrology	Respiratory
Neurology and Electro-	Services/PFT
diagnostic	Nuclear Medicine
Medical Education	Physical Therapy

Rehabilitation	Neonatal Units
Medicine	Burn Units
Hematology/Blood-	Immunology Laboratory
clotting Laboratory	

The schismatic process has not yet been completed, and further budding is likely.

Under the current social structure, the physician is the only person on the hospital's team licensed to practice medicine. Since most of the departments enumerated above have a major impact on the practice of medicine within the hospital, a medical director is a legal necessity if a department is to be utilized effectively for the benefit of the hospital, its patients, and its medical staff. The problem is that a director can assume as much or as little of the requisite function as he wishes. This is so because of limitations of medical practice; most hospitals tend formally or informally to act as if the physician were an independent contractor. Almost uniformly, physicians are neither trained nor prepared, during their specialty training, for a managerial role. Thus the physician appointed as director, when confronted with an apparently insoluble problem, can easily retreat into the fastness of his patient care activities or his technical services to escape from the pressures generated in his department.

The hospital provides these independent contracting physicians with vast arrays of complex facilities, sometimes with thousands of square feet and dozens of hospital employees to direct. Unfortunately, most of the new departments mentioned above have yet to develop stable, adequate supplies of trained paramedical talent. The newer the department the greater the demand placed upon its medical director. The director must not only manage the medical portion of his department's activities but also upgrade his assistants and conduct an on-the-job training program to meet increasing departmental demands as they develop.

Since very likely the only training the director has had in this area is watching his "chief" during the course of his training period, in activities whose significance he is only now realizing, this will present some added stress.

Another unanticipated pressure upon the medical director is that most of the above-named departments are on the hospital's list of income producers. The implication is that the director must maintain the income-producing capacity of his department and even augment it by applying his superior specialty training. At the very least, he is expected not to impede the department's income-producing functions. That constraint is particularly onerous; for the young director may have blithely assumed that his sole requirement would be to exercise the technical medical skills taught him at his postgraduate institution. Unfortunately, his technical skills and the income production of his department are not directly related. He may come under additional stress when he learns that his position is coveted by others with an equal amount of training and it is therefore doubly expedient for him to produce in the expected fashion. His simple world has suddenly become highly complex. If he is not up on the rules in the fast ballgame, he may be called out or put back on the bench.

While he tries to satisfy the medical staff, the administration, the patients, and his own departmental staff, the medical director may also find that certain areas of his department's activities are in danger of being split off to form new subdepartments under other directors. The discipline once simply called pathology has now evolved, for example, into a potentially separate activity called forensic medicine as well as a major subcategory known as clinical laboratory sciences. While there is not much further schismatic tendency in pathology and forensic medicine, there is in the laboratory sciences. Already arterial blood gases, once a province of the clinical laboratory specialist, has been moved over to a new discipline—the department of Respiratory Services. On the horizon are similar tendencies to split off specialized hematological procedures, immunological procedures, gastrointestinal titration procedures, and the radioimmuno-assays of various biological products. The same tendency toward reproduction by fission is present in many of the other "regular departments." Cardiology was once merely a service for the reading of the electrocardiogram with an affiliated consulting service. It has now grown to such a point that a large number of services requiring highly specialized training have developed; they include noninvasive cardiac diagnosis (phonocardiogram, echocardiogram, and so on) and invasive cardiac diagnostic methods (cardiac catheterization). In addition, a new subset of clinical cardiology labeled coronary care units and progressive coronary care units are evolving and requiring specialized attention and medical direction. Finally, cardiac rehabilitation programs may also require some director's time and attention in the future.

The overall picture is complicated still further by the 16 to 17 percent increase, over the past ten years, in the number of persons exceeding age 65. The significance of this demographic fact to hospital departments is that this elderly age group has become the most avid consumer of health services. The growing number of elderly has had a tremendous impact upon hospital utilization, since most of these people have chronic processes requiring multiple health services. Previously hospitals were planned and built to take care of the acutely and temporarily ill with predominantly self-limited processes. The major shift in population has resulted in a major change in the spectrum of illnesses presented to the hospital. Evidently that has been overlooked by the majority of health planners who have input into medical school curricula and into planning for new hospital services.

The current fact of life is that chronic recurrent disease with acute exacerbation is or will soon become the predominant disease entity in the hospital. Directors who have been specifically trained to differentiate between the acutely ill and the chronically ill with exacerbations will be the ones to react most appropriately. The result will be improved and more efficient utilization of their services, but the price will be the increased demand upon them to personally tutor or otherwise educate the medical staff into differentiating between the therapeutic approaches necessary in treating the acutely ill as contrasted with the acute exacerbation of the chronically ill. This merely adds another layer to the tasks of the medical director.

Thus the director finds himself, instead of stepping into a position in which he can concentrate upon doing things in which he has been specifically trained, engulfed in a great amount of human in-

teraction, public relations, and other management functions—
activities that he never expected and certainly never anticipated.
Many physicians will resent this constraint of social pressures that
they feel is manipulated to make them jump neatly through the
hospital's hoops.

THE COST CRISIS IN HEALTH CARE

The problem of the demand for further services and
the emphasis on the earning of money in the department is usually
compounded by the administrator's constant cry, "I can't give you
what you need to do the job." In fact, the whole country is demanding cheaper health care at the same time that it is demanding
better and more elaborate health services. Obviously, this burden
of satisfying the demand for more with less will be skillfully diverted by the hospital administration to the medical directors of the
various departments. The real problem is that people are no longer
dying quietly at home and without incurring too great a cost in
health care. With increased longevity and the demand for a better
quality of life as well as health, we have now reached the point
where many more patients are being readmitted to hospitals and,
more significantly, are ultimately dying in those hospitals.

However much we might like to give everyone the ultimate in
care, the fact is that we cannot afford to give everyone the ultimate
in care. The directors of specialty departments are in the best positions to notice overutilization; for they see the same pattern of ad-
missions and treatments day in and day out and so can recognize
trends as, for example, in the field of cardiology. Thirty years ago
the mortality from the acute myocardial infarction was approxi-
mately 40 percent; today it is about 20 percent. This represents a
very significant salvage in life, but the problem is that there has
been a twentyfold increase in cost. If cardiac catheterization and
coronary artery bypass surgery are added to the therapeutic
modalities for this illness, there is probably an additional tenfold
increase in cost.

To make matters worse, the more successful you are in salvaging lives, the more utilization you insure yourself: the patients you have saved from dying now are likely to return later. If you are successful in prolonging life long enough, most patients admitted to the hospitals will have two or more major system involvements. Each may require the services of a subspecialist and his or her department. Again, the utilization factor goes up, but whether the quality-of-life factor improves at all is debatable. This is obviously an explosive growth situation in which no one can decry taking each specific therapeutic action even though the overall costs are mounting horrendously. With the doubling in number of people over 65, one can predict a very busy time indeed for every active medical director.

Since the hospital receives a major share of its reimbursement for this older age group from public funds, the problem of compliance with bureaucratic regulations becomes paramount. In many cases, the people who are in charge of government policy and the third-party insurance payers are totally removed from the immediate clinical problem upon which their directives bear so importantly. If, as is usual, they are planning for circumstances that are ten or fifteen years in the past, their regulations and codes are inappropriate to the current situation. And although the U.S. judicial system is based upon English common law, most bureaucratic regulations are philosophically based upon the Napoleonic Code: you are presumed guilty until you have proved yourself innocent.

The consequence is that the hospital and its medical directors are required to prove that they are indeed providing appropriate and relevant services to public patients. If the guidelines and regulations laid down by some civil servant physician, who is probably many years removed from actual direct medical care, are inappropriate to the present situation, then the dilemma of increased demand for services is augmented by the question of who will pay for the necessary documentation of need. The director may have to evolve some method whereby the hospital can obtain reimbursement for services it provides even though the regulations do not admit of such services. This gives the director a crisis of conscience. Does he in effect lie and give the patient the treatment he needs and insure that the hospital receives the money it needs, or does he tilt with windmills in trying to convince some distant bureaucrat that he doesn't know what is going on?

Ten years ago it became apparent to the medical community that the number of patients with chronic respiratory diseases was rapidly increasing. A large number of chest physicians and directors who had to deal with these patients recognized that the patients required education in preventive measures so that they would at least not aggravate their pathophysiological processes. The efforts initially were either *sub rosa* or nonexistent. Now, a decade later, the government's reimbursement policy has finally been broadened by the admission that there are indeed chronically ill patients in the community for whom education may be appropriate. The department just might pay for such educational services as part of the treatment modality if the prescribed format is followed.

Unfortunately, that does nothing for the first decade's crop of patients who could have benefited by a shorter lag time to the development of a more appropriate therapeutic and reimbursement policy. The lesson is that the medical director can anticipate that health regulations will be out of phase with clinical reality by months, if not years. He will have to try to meet the needs of his specialty, satisfy his hospital, and comply with the paperwork regulations of government agencies, all in keeping with the practice of good medicine.

In addition to all this, the government is now saying it can no longer continue to pay costs as determined by the health care provider; instead, it must have an estimate to which the physician and the hospital will rigidly adhere. This is much the same policy change that occurred in the 1960s in the aerospace industry. In the words of Henry X. Jackson, "hospitals are now sliding into a capital crunch." The government has decided it can no longer afford to pay for all the care the patients are getting and has therefore tried to opt out by paying only the direct costs incurred by patients for whom it is responsible.

That may be an ideal accounting procedure for someone trying to escape paying his fair share by limiting his liability to current services and disclaiming any responsibility for the equipment, capital investments, personnel training, and standby facilities that are required. But it is clearly a short-term policy. Ultimately someone else will have to pay for the maintenance of present services, replacement of services as necessary, and development of new services; otherwise, the services will deteriorate. To have that occur while another branch of government is insisting upon increasing adherence to high levels of health care standards is doubly contradictory. And since the hospital has already laid the burden of maintaining the earnings of the department on his shoulders, the director will be in the forefront of the battle. He will find that he is involved in the politics of medical health care and health care payment whether he wishes to be or not.

Directors of the various departments may find it essential to work together to develop policies permitting the type of patient care necessary within the constraints laid upon them by the Department of Health, Education and Welfare and others. In southern California recently, a group effort was made over five years to get the government medical plan amended to provide pulmonary rehabilitation for chronic pulmonary patients. Such patients had been repeatedly demonstrated to be very high consumers of health care, and the cost of acute exacerbations was becoming excessively high. Now, after only five years, which may be a record time, an unofficial pilot program to meet this need is in the process of development. Thus the medical directors involved can probably stop providing bootleg rehabilitation services and go legal, but the same problem will continue to exist for other directors with similar needs.

DIRECTOR QUALIFICATIONS AND BACKGROUND

Perhaps the preceding remarks give the impression that the first requirement of the medical director is that he be a close relative of Superman. Failing that, he must become superorganized to handle all of the diverse functions that he never imagined he would be involved in. And, since a major function is to adapt widely varying patient demands to a relatively inflexible health care plan, he must have a ready facility for dealing with people and paper and for withstanding stress.

Amazingly, the Joint Commission on Accreditation of Hospitals has specified formal training requirements only for directors of Pathology and Radiology.[3] Their training requirements for Anesthesia, Emergency Room, Outpatient Services, Nuclear Medicine, Physical Medicine, Respiratory Diseases, and Special Care Units are very general. Evidently requirements in these areas are to be determined by the medical staff bylaws and regulations. In the areas not even mentioned by implication, the path to directorship is totally dependent upon local tastes and circumstances.

Thus in most instances there are multiple paths toward a directorship. Ultimately, of course, the requirements will depend to a great degree upon the sophistication and experience of the medical staff of the particular hospital. However, in the less formal situations the physician's previous training may have less to do with his qualifications for the position than his current activities, interests, and demonstrated abilities and, most importantly, his contacts. The scene can be expected to change rapidly, however, since most government agencies will soon require the captain to have a master's certificate. Where older physicians are in charge (under the grandfather clause), even though they have a wealth of experience, they are likely to be under increasing pressure to take aboard someone with a pilot's license.

Although the Joint Commission regards medical directors as highly necessary and even essential to the operation of some of the hospital's specialty departments, the medical staff generally is not of that opinion. Hospital medical staffs tend to believe that the director's position is just a soft, cushy administrative job and therefore bureaucratically wasteful. Medical staff physicians can appreciate the hospital-based doctor only when he provides their own patients with an appropriate service.

The challenge by certain elements of the hospital medical staff is that a person, if adequately trained in his own specialty, should be able to do his own specialty diagnostic interpretation. Essentially, the medical staff has missed the point that the medical director does far more than merely read diagnostic tests each day. The other side of the coin is that there are in fact any number of bad medical directors such as those who have subcontracted services to young physicians and are, in effect, absentee landlords. Certainly such people tend to keep alive the bitterness and resentment that are so easily fanned in times of stress.

Unfortunately, there is nothing in the medical school curriculum about the function of the director of a department, so most graduate M.D.'s are largely ignorant of any but the obvious technical aspects of the position. Doctors who are aiming for directorship positions, therefore, not only suffer from lack of training but also, because their colleagues are ignorant of the management functions that they need to perform, lack the stimulus of informed peer expectation. Most directors pick up their management skills by a weird process of osmosis and apprenticeship. While in training they may notice their chief in his more obvious activities, and they tend to adopt the more visible portions of his approach without realizing that what is valid for Doctor A in Institution B may be totally inappropriate for Doctor C in Institution D. Until the Joint Commission requires some evidence of formal management training in the undergraduate years, such training is likely to be based more upon the principle of the survival of the fittest than upon management by objectives.

NONMEDICAL MANAGEMENT FUNCTIONS

The varieties of formal functions that the director will probably have to perform are described in some detail in Chapters 2 to 4, but there are other and less obvious functions as well. These irregular aspects of management are as essential to the director's performance as a foundation is to a house. They will never be mentioned either in the director's contract or in his discussions with the chief executive officer of the hospital. The functions that are hinted at but never openly discussed are as follows:

1. Leader and strategic planner
2. Promoter and producer
3. Salesmanager
4. Quality and product control officer
5. Reformer and showman
6. Public relations man
7. Report writer
8. Intelligence agent
9. On-demand competitor

The first such function is that of *leadership*. Perhaps no one finds it necessary to discuss this function, precisely because it is so obvious. Certainly there are decisions, policies, and responses that need to be made almost every day in the course of activities of a department. If the director is not there often enough, someone else will begin to make the necessary decisions. Thus the medical director, even though he is the sole possessor of the medical license in his department, cannot anticipate freedom of decision if he is not available to the department on a sufficiently continuous basis to exert the leadership that is implicit in his position as director.

In the director's absence, especially in clinical departments, certain departmental personnel will respond and react in their own way at their own level. They may begin to feel, and often with considerable justification, that they could perform just as well without the director. The director's salvation lies in the fact that there is so much that he can do that the paramedical staff can never replace or even compete with. Nevertheless, in a number of instances the subsidiary personnel of a department have been successful in forcing out a difficult director who paid too little attention to leadership. Leadership and absenteeism are incompatible.

The second of the *sub rosa* functions is the director's role as a *promoter* and *sales manager* of his department. Each time a clinical pathological conference is made more interesting by findings from a new laboratory or radiological procedure, the speaker is promoting the procedure's use. The problem with promotion is that most medical directors become aware of it only when a new piece of equipment becomes available. What the director must realize is that he must examine and analyze the modes of utilization of his department, identify deficiencies in utilization or in the indications for the particular test, and proceed subtly to promote a more proper or more adequate method of utilization. He will undoubtedly find that what he wants to promote is more effective utilization of the mainstays of his department, because that is where most people tend to be lax. They are too interested in the unusual and the unique to pay attention to what is commonplace. If the director can improve utilization of tests that are done on a daily basis, the return is far greater than from something that is ordered once or twice a year.

One of the most inobvious *sub rosa* functions of the medical director is his educational activity. A professor usually finds his students as receptive to his words as baby robins are to the mother bringing back the food. But out in the community, the gradient between your knowledge and the staff physician's is less obvious (to the medical staff, that is), and the automatic flow of knowledge from director to medical staff may not occur in the absence of appropriate planning. (See the discussion on the U.S. consultant versus European tradition in Chapter 8.) The medical director's most effective teaching occurs not in a formal setting, but rather in a one-to-one relationship in which he and a physician are looking at a particular problem and deciding how to handle it. The same one-to-one training must occur with each paramedical technician and nurse with whom the director comes into contact in the hospital.

The problem is that most people stop learning as soon as they step out of a situation labeled school. Thus the date of a physician's departure from his training institution is probably that of a substantial fraction of his techniques, applications, and work-ups. You, as a newer graduate, may find that the clinician not only exhibits ignorance of the newer techniques but also is likely to resist learning a new technique because he is not in a "training situation." Learning about things that you do not know exist is difficult when you are not prepared to admit the new information.

With the enactment of Public Law 92-603, and with the deterioration in the malpractice situation, it has become almost mandatory that some sort of peer review surveillance and upgrading activity be conducted in your hospital on a regular basis. The Joint Commission has initiated this change of affairs, and much of it can still be adapted to with sheer paperwork from the committees and have little impact upon the medical staff's activities, patterns, and habits. That, however, is true only of the first time around; if you are to be effective over the long term, you will need to change the medical staff's basic approaches to what has previously been done in a less than optimal fashion.

In this program of self-help, the peer review can be a golden opportunity for the medical director. Previously it would have been impossible to direct so much attention to routine care patterns that may have had built into them tremendous amounts of error. There is quite a philosophical battle going on over whether continuing education should be mandatory. In the meantime, however, you had best confine your teaching activities to regular *sub rosa* efforts on a one-to-one basis. Ability to subtly provide information to another physician is what will make your reputation as an esteemed clinician in the long run.

Another major *sub rosa* function is that of public relations. You must use public relations and all the management skills already discussed in working with your own team to make sure that it meshes with the larger hospital team. You set the tenor and tone of your department by your own performance. If you are pessimistic, curt, and sullen, you undoubtedly will have people who will emulate you. If you are a bubbling, effervescent type of person, you are more likely to spark a similar demeanor in your staff. You really should assess yourself in this regard to ascertain whether your approach to life will affect the type of personnel your department will attract.

The number of solvent negativistic public relations people is probably quite small. The occupation tends to attract those who are positive and reasonably outgoing. If those traits are not native to you, they can be acquired, since your interest in other people is not synthetic or phoney but is actually quite rational and real. Obviously if your team must perform some critical function during an emergency, it behooves you to know that the other hospital people also perform their functions satisfactorily. Thus their attitude, philosophy, and training are important because you and they are all in the same ship. The public relations function is not one of selling your department as a department; rather it is selling the idea that you and your people must get along with and work with the others. That is actually far more difficult to sell than a concrete piece of equipment or a specific delineated service.

A final *sub rosa* function, one that, again, is rarely mentioned because it is so often taken for granted, is the *writing of reports*. If you write reports only once a year when the budget comes due, you will probably hamper your career and your department considerably. Hospital administrations operate on paper (Chapter 4). Therefore, you must generate your fair share of the appropriate paperwork to meet your commitments to the hospital and to the third-party payers. Finally, Peer Review, the Joint Commission, Audit, and Quality Control will also require written records, so there really is no way to escape the necessity for paperwork. One can, of course, force the task upon someone at a lower level, but then the performance also may be lower.

The best time to begin writing reports is when you first visit an institution in which you have an interest. You need immediately to write a response to the administration and detail what it is you have in mind. You want the reader to come inescapably to the conclusions that you have planned for, namely, that here is a well-organized and direct person who can plan intelligently and is worth talking to again. You will have further exposure to report writing subsequently, but the function begins with your preliminary letter of inquiry and response to replies.

THE PATIENT'S PHYSICIAN AS PURCHASING AGENT

One of the realities that again may be labeled *sub rosa* is the variety of ways in which you can look at your major customer, the primary care physician. Each physician in practice has hundreds or thousands of patients for whom he has responsibility.

In the process of following them and caring for them he can utilize either Product A or Product B for many common conditions. Pharmaceutical companies long ago recognized the potentialities of the situation and have concentrated tremendous amounts of money and effort upon convincing physicians that their Product A is superior to someone else's Product B. They realize that if you can convince one doctor that A is better than B, he may prescribe A tens, hundreds, or thousands of times a year. Therefore, their approach to the primary physician is that he is acting as a purchasing agent for a group of patients.

That same realization should become part of the medical director's armamentarium. Even though Doctor X admits only twenty-five patients to your hospital each year, if you can show him how to order the work-up for the common conditions in an appropriate and useful manner, you will undoubtedly find that the utilization of procedures will increase. If you have properly instructed Doctor X, his work-up and consequently his treatment of his patient will be that much improved.

In addition to possibly obtaining far greater improvement in medical care indirectly than you could directly, you will find that the indirect approach of necessity changes the way you handle physicians. Obviously, they are no longer merely your peers, or competitors, but people with tremendous power as well. Thus you are less likely to insult or put down one of them because of some misuse or ill-use of a modality. There is a proverb that says, "Oh Lord, give me balance of mind that I may not utter sharp words today that I will have to eat tomorrow." It is particularly pertinent to this problem, since doctors are on such an elevated plane of ego development that they do not take off-the-cuff criticism at all well. So a corollary to your treating the primary physician as a purchasing agent is another *sub rosa* talent: you must keep your hospital medical staff happy and satisfied with your department.

Again, I do not believe you'll find that in any contract, and probably not in any discussion with an administrator either. Legally you could insult every physician to such an extent that he would stop using your department and still be within your contractual obligation. However, the practical result would be a very short period of service to your ego, since the position you occupied would undoubtedly evaporate with its doctor-client population. Thus you must reorder your goals: you must stop being right and instead become effective.

DEPARTMENTAL INTEGRATION WITH
THE TOTAL HOSPITAL EFFORT

In this day of subspecialty training it is difficult sometimes to see the forest for the tree you are most interested in. However, to point out the obvious, it will not make a bit of difference to patient care if your department is the best in the world if it is unable to operate in concert with the rest of the hospital. There may be situations in which it is necessary for you to pull in your horns so that another department also can operate effectively; otherwise, you may destroy a vital balance that is essential to teamwork. That balance may be in terms of logistics, supply, floor area, morale, or personnel. The importance of the balance is proportional to the importance of your department in the hospital. If you direct a small department with a minimal range of services, it is not likely that your total cooperation will be crucial to many patients. But if you direct a major department that interacts with most of the hospital and if you set a tone of aloofness, separateness, and competition, the ones who will suffer will be the patients.

Everyone gives lip service to the proposition that meeting patient needs requires cooperation, give and take, and coordination of activities. Taking a portable chest x-ray for endotracheal tube position before the tube has been inserted is hardly optimum coordination. Similarly, transporting patients who require oxygen without oxygen, or performing unnecessarily repeated blood sampling procedures on critically ill patients, would also indicate poor interdepartmental cooperation. In each instance it is the patient who ultimately suffers, but somewhere along the line departmental reputations also may be blemished.

One particularly pernicious instance of poor interdepartmental cooperation occurs when a diagnostic service locks up all its records and tests when the chief of the department and the medical director are absent. Any physician who wishes to look up some vital piece of information becomes totally frustrated. The disadvantage to the department head, of course, is that the doctor may learn to do without the department's services altogether.

Individual strategies to break down some of these barriers are so personal and so related to the Gestalt of the particular situation that generalities about them are hardly of any use. It is worth noting, however, that if you as a director are relatively noncompetitive, and if you are pitted against a group of competitive departments, you will not be able to hold your own unless you learn to be somewhat competitive yourself. After all, the welfare of your patients is at stake. So when other departments are taking precedence in capital investment, staffing, and so on, you can either fight to regain your fair share or else allow your department to be slowly ground away to an ineffectual nub. Administrators keep a very close eye on the balance sheet of each department's financial activities. If your department's services or charges are gradually being whittled away, the chief executive officer will be quick to notice.

The problem of competition for space, time, and services may be complicated by the open or covert jealousy that the hospital-based physician encounters in his medical staff peers. Such jealousy commonly results in preposterous demands for services. Most hospital staff physicians do their rounds early in the morning and expect that, between the time they arrive and write an order and the time they go to their offices, the procedures ordered will have been completed and reported on the chart. Now if a physician orders a multiplicity of urgent tests to be performed on a given patient, it is fairly obvious that only a few of the total can be accomplished in that time. So if you find your department has been blasted for nonperformance of a service but scrutiny of the chart reveals there was no way all of the services ordered could have been performed in the time allowed, you have warning that someone is out after you.

If the preceding medical director is still on the staff, you may find him to be an additional source of jealousy. Historically, hospital departments often have highly informal origins. The leading local expert in the field is selected to act as voluntary director. At some point in time it is obvious to both administration and medical staff, and quite often to the incumbent himself, that he cannot give enough time to the department without giving up all of his own private patients. It is best when the voluntary director is the first to realize this and to understand that he has an option either to direct full time after getting additional training or, as he more often prefers, to bring in an outside person so he can keep his practice-based option open.

In either case, you may not have the major jealousy problem you have when the incumbent is forced out by concerted action of the medical staff and administration because of his inadequacies. However, there are many people who, having started something, regard it as their own and cannot give it up. That is true of parents with children, and it is true of first directors of departments. Even though a first director was a prime mover in bringing you in, he may be a continuing source of irritation as you try to change the method of operation. Add to that the realization by the voluntary physician that he did all this extra work for nothing, whereas you, the official hospital-based physician, are receiving reasonable remuneration, and you may ultimately see some raised hackles that no one ever thought existed.

INTERDEPARTMENTAL COMPETITION FOR INCOME

In addition to the minor factional disputes and individual jealousies referred to above, a more important issue is that of cutting up the pie of patient services and disposing of the pieces. You may have a departmental responsibility that is well defined with clear boundaries, or yours may be an area in which the responsibility for services is a matter of opinion instead of cold, clear logic. Consequently, you may be either the recipient of someone else's interest in invading your field or the one who is invading another field in an attempt to develop it along a different line. In either instance, as the pie grows larger, the boundaries become less well defined and the question of where a particular service goes becomes vital.

When pulmonary specialists were rare, many departments were started up as cardiopulmonary services because cardiologists did possess some pulmonary expertise. When personnel with specific pulmonary training became available, those departments were sometimes split. The new pulmonary departments then proceeded to aggrandize activities from the general laboratory for arterial blood gases. Further areas of growth may be back into the field of cardiology with the Swann-Ganz catheter technique or into surgical fields by endoscopic procedures with biopsy techniques.

The same kind of development is true of other clinical departments that have grown into the new field of fiber optic endoscopy, as well as a totally different area such as that of diagnostic ultrasound. In the latter instance the technique could be used with equal facility by Neurology, Cardiology, Radiology, and Nuclear Medicine. Each department protests that it can do a better job than the others. The struggle for control of ultrasound will depend upon the personalities and backgrounds of the directors involved.

The concept of a single hospital machine shared equally among several departments is rather inappropriate for the reason that led to the established separate departments in the first place. From a purely financial point of view, you must have a department and a departmental organization so that services can be charged for properly, equipment can be maintained and serviced, and staffing and personnel can be adjusted to the needs of the hospital. Certainly in the case of ultrasound, staffing provided by one department may be quite different from that provided by another, so that the accessibility of this service may be determined by the resources of the other department and its directors.

All too often the more senior department with the more extensive political connections manages to take over the new service even though the technique may be just as appropriate to another discipline. In instances in which the conflict is rather brisk and facts exist to support each department's arguments, a hospital may try to solve the problem by buying each department its own machine. It thus absorbs the additional capital expense itself; for certainly no government agency would approve of such extravagance as a double coverage of a single service.

Currently there are numerous areas that interact and encroach upon one another. Most of them revolve around the clinical diagnostic departments. Presently there is a new technological development of continuous in-line monitoring of blood gases. These techniques could be used equally well by the departments of Anesthesiology, Cardiology, and Respiratory Services. Although all have good arguments for possessing the machine, in most instances only one department will get it; and whatever department gets the machine will have an edge over the others in terms of bargaining for further improvements. So the battle progresses.

If a director should allow too many other departments to take away services that he might potentially offer, his departmental income will drop and so will the stability of his position. Thus, in general, a director is not going to willingly give up any modality that might have a significant impact upon his department's economic future. The only way he can afford to give up a modality is by arranging a trade or by developing a substitute source of service and income.

A recent example in point had to do with blood gases. The Joint Commission on Accreditation of Hospitals recommended that arterial blood gas determinations be performed by Respiratory Services, since the personnel of that department are specifically trained to use the information generated in their clinical activities. Thus maximal efficiency in a rapidly changing clinical situation is assured by placing the entire feedback loop within the involved department. But since arterial blood gas determinations had been an income producer for the hospital departments running them, some sort of trade-off was necessary.

Sometimes the director can become involved in such trade-offs by helping to assure the department losing the service that the loss is short-term only. If, for example, respiratory care is improved, then the number of patients surviving will increase and the utiliza-

tion of other departmental services by the survivors also will increase. Obviously, the director must become highly skilled politically in order to effect a smooth transition with no open battles.

THE NECESSITY FOR PLANNING

The most openly accepted and well-defined task of
each director is planning for the future. But although everyone
agrees that planning is necessary and the director is the man to do
it, most directors proceed on a day-to-day basis. That may be because so many directors have had no management, administrative,
or executive training. Certainly once you have assumed responsibility for a department, you need to be responsible not only for day-
to-day activities but for long-term policies as well.

Most directors, however, seem to rely much too heavily upon
demands from the attending medical staff for signals as to what
they should do next. To paraphrase one conversation, a director
stated that he is problem-oriented rather than goal-oriented. That
is, he remains in a state of leadership stasis until a problem arises.
He then attempts to solve the problem to the satisfaction of himself
and other concerned parties. Following that, he returns to the state
of ready reserve while he awaits the next problem. In contrast, the
goal-oriented director deduces from past and current evidence what
trends are likely and what changes will be needed, and he has the
changes available as the needs become obvious and urgent.

One of the underlying reasons for the lack of long-term
strategic activity by the director may be the basic division between
administration and the hospital-based physician. While the administrator may speak glowingly to each new director about planning
the future together, the medical director soon learns that what that
really means is that the administrator plans their future together
with little or no input from the medical director. He may, when he
feels so inclined, ask for technical help, but he looks to others for
guidance in determining future areas of service. In many instances,
the director's first notice that something new is afoot is when he
receives reports that an outside planning agency has completed a

survey in the hospital, usually without ever questioning him. He then is presented with the recommendations and asked to consider their impact upon the department's future activities and discuss the consequences with the administration. Events such as these merely reinforce the director's tendency to minimize his problems by dealing only with those that are immediate and resolvable at his level.

Directors who do attempt to plan their own long-term future must learn to use the hospital medical staff as a support force and camouflage. If after due consideration and deliberation, the medical director decides that plan A is a high-priority option that should be available, he will, if he is politically sophisticated, try to enlist power groups to cosponsor his plan. Otherwise, the administrator could always argue and say, "Well, I have other important things to consider first."

What the director should do is approach the more amenable among the prominent and appropriate staff physicians and convince them of the need for the new step. Only then is plan A considered for presentation to the administration. This approach has its disadvantages, of course. The power group proposing the plan may not be fully aware of its intricacies, and so you must be included in the presentation. True planning among equals requires assessment and evaluation of the current position, the future needs that must be met, and the other factors that might influence events. To carry any weight in this type of game you must have adequate information about what is going on in other important areas in the hospital. But that requires much more ready access to administrative levels of information and control than most medical directors appear to have.

The essential issue in long-term planning, then, is to learn who is who in terms of decision making and who has input to the decision makers, both in the institution and locally in the community. Unless you can tap into a line that is receptive to your data, analysis of the facts, and proposals, you are better off not even trying, except as a training exercise for your own education. You must be able to look at your proposal with the eyes of the hospital administrator and try to ascertain which of its aspects would most excite hostility and counteraggression as well as approval. Obviously, to consider your proposals in that light, you need to have considerable preparation that includes a review by persons who can give you an independent opinion as to the probable value of the proposals.

At this point the question that arises is whether you should discuss your plan with your peer medical directors in the hospital. Most directors are not too concerned with larger, long-range problems; they expect to receive adequate warning of needed changes from someone else on the staff. From that point of view it should not be too difficult to find out what people want, because most of them don't want anything except to just keep putting one foot in front of the other. However, that represents only one side of the issue; for if you concretely and specifically try to include the other hospital-based physicians in your survey of potential trends, you will quickly find some who are ready to act as spoilers. They immediately recognize the challenge you present by being interested in what is going to happen instead of taking a passive attitude. Thus they will offer counterplans whose effect may be calculated as much to stall your plans as to meet any other real needs in the future. In a competition for resources for major services in the future, giving advance notice of your intent to sequester some of the funds may promote a capital frenzy not unlike the feeding frenzy of sharks.

So it may be best not to share your innermost long-range speculations with other medical directors too early. At some point you must inform the others, since they are part of the power group that will have to acquiesce in your proposal. One way to do so is to wait until your plans are so well developed that any counterproposal would appear ludicrously sketchy and ineffective in contrast. A more positive approach is first to ascertain the impact your plans will have on other departments and then approach the heads of those departments with which the interface is significant with proposals for codevelopment of their departments' activities as well as yours. By acquainting them with developments that they may not have been aware of, you may engender a groundswell of support for the total proposal.

That is simply a practical matter of getting some solid, reliable political allies so that, when you have your plan ready for presentation, someone will do you the favor of supporting it. Obviously, elements of self-interest are intrinsic to this approach, since your getting a major portion of limited hospital capital resources means that other departments will have a smaller part of the pie to share. Accordingly, their directors will expect some compensatory benefits. Yours is not a hypocritical gesture of buying votes but a solidly practical one of making certain that what you are planning has benefit to more than a very limited number of doctors and patients. Since any number of growth areas are available to each department, your concerned interest in someone else's future, particularly when it melds well with yours, is appreciated.

Of course, none of the preceding remarks on planning may have much relevance if the administrator exercises absolute power over the direction his hospital takes. It is in those situations that you must use the demands of the medical staff as both a shield and a tactical weapon. No matter how dictatorial an administrator is, he knows that the independent members of his medical staff, the primary care physicians, are totally free to take their patients to any hospital they like. Logically he should not engage in open conflict with them because they can pick up their pieces and move the game. He can, of course, manage the few physicians that he controls directly, but he has no power to fill his hospital except by the good graces of the primary care physicians in his community. Those considerations would be unnecessary if the administrator were openly receptive to input from all of his medical directors and from the medical staff as well.

THE IMPORTANCE OF SIZING UP THE ADMINISTRATOR

Some administrators are genuinely open to input from the medical staff; others are middle-of-the-road people who know what they want but do try to gain a consensus and are willing to amend their plans to meet the wishes and needs of others; and then there are the feudal lords who look upon hospitals as their fiefs and medical directors as their vassals. It should be apparent that you must quickly divine the administrative philosophy of the hospital in which you are interested. Once you have arrived, signed a contract, become established, and made financial commitments, it is rather late to find out that you cannot live and work effectively under the prevailing circumstances. The deed is done; you are committed; and the easiest thing for you to do then is adapt, since certainly the administrator will not. That is probably why so many medical directors quickly assume a passive posture. So if you have ideals that cannot easily be shaped by external pressures and events, you had best very quickly determine the mood and the philosophy of any institution with which you are considering long-term affiliation.

Since the administrator deals so intimately with the medical staff, his philosophy usually has its exact counterpart in that of the medical staff. Merely by virtue of the power his superior position insures, the administrator tends to have chiefs of staff who are sympathetic with his philosophy and can work comfortably with him. The problem the young physician faces is how to determine all these highly intangible but crucially important factors in a few brief visits. The best way is to pose a few key questions. One of these is who makes the decisions when the administrator is away. If no decisions are made until he returns, and if in addition he is away frequently, be alerted to the possibility of an absolutist type of administration that might be very uncomfortable in the long term.

A question to ask the existing medical directors is how involved they are, on a yearly basis, with the administration in planning the course of their various departments. If the answer is nonspecific, ask for an estimate of how many hours they spend in developing plans and presenting them to administration. If the number of hours quoted is near zero, it is obvious that this is a Captain Queeg type of operation that may or may not fit in with your plans. If, in addition, most of the medical directors are unaware of what is going on in other departments, you may be sure the administrator is using the powers of secrecy and competition to divide and conquer.

If you are frustrated at your present hospital level, there are some other political resources that you may be able to tap. Every administrator recognizes the benefits of good public relations and is quite pleased to have his hospital's reputation enhanced in the community. If you can develop any activity that involves community support and that ultimately brings more patients to the hospital, you may by your very success become important enough for your plans to be given some consideration. Also, if the opportunity presents itself, you may visit other hospitals to see if a position might be open for you elsewhere either then or in the future to give you a more secure power base. But in doing all this you are skating near the edge and must be aware that some of your activities may be supportive and others may be directly threatening to the administrator. The only way to find out is to see what response he will make.

2

THE
MANAGEMENT
FUNCTION

THE NEED FOR MANAGEMENT SKILLS

As professionals, physicians have great pride in their status and tend to react emotionally rather than search for causes when unanticipated career derailments occur. A recent study[4] showed, among 50 hospital positions observed, a 68 percent turnover rate in five years that could be attributed to management, not technical, problems. Among their peers, the conversation of the holders of such positions was restricted to current clinical problems and successes; thus no advantage was taken of an opportunity to gain insight into the problems responsible for the high turnover rate.

Extensive samplings of a wider range of hospital-based specialties revealed a similar pattern of career changes. The traditional specialties, pathology, radiology, and anesthesiology, were the most stable. Presumably the long period of apprenticeship before attaining the top posts and the extensive standard operating procedures served to carry most young directors through management problems. However, the directors from fields lacking either a well-established operational code or a long period of apprenticeship had as their major concerns in private conversations the entire gamut of management problems.

The increasing complexity of the current health system has served to intensify the already great need for management skills among physicians in leadership positions. Yet such training and experience are absent in both medical school curricula and specialty training programs. The professional literature on this subject is scanty and superficial, so that the questing physician is without any coherent information resources. The entire orientation of physician training is to develop a uniquely skilled professional who needs little help to accomplish his task—in effect there seems to be an antimanagement bias throughout it.

Today's hospitals are complex organizations with increasing demands for participation by and contributions from physician–medical directors in the attainment of various departmental goals. An organization is an entity that coordinates a large number of people to perform explicitly defined tasks to reach objectives that the individual cannot reach alone. Hospitals as organizations have a varied number of departments that differ in their characteristics and goals. But all hospitals have basic essential qualities such as rationality of purpose and need for effective performance and fiscal efficiency in the achievement of their departmental and total hospital goals. More to that point is the following quotation:[5]

> More and more professions are being pursued in bureaucratic settings. Even for the physician and the lawyer, the last of the "free professionals," practice is increasingly a group enterprise, boxed in with various organizational constraints. Private practice as a style of professional work is rapidly waning/disappearing; many new and emergent professions/specialties have never practiced in anything except a bureaucratic setting.

MANAGEMENT FUNCTIONS

When we speak about management in the field of medicine, we refer to those nontechnical activities that should be performed by the "leader" of the department. Ideally, the leader should be a physician. However, the role is tied not to the M.D. degree, but to a function, namely, that of organizing and coordinating the activities of a varied number of health personnel through cooperative means and direct action toward the attainment of a common goal.

To manage, you must be able to control. Consequently, the manager must know what *authority* he possesses to perform his function. Thus the manager will make decisions the nature of which will be affected by the demands of the environment, the institution, and his particular department. In that role he will be acting as the leader and should be using his decision-making powers in accord with the overall management policy of the hospital to achieve his portion of the total goal. To achieve his goal he must set objectives, both short- and long-term. A subfunction of objective setting is the constraint to be realistic. The objectives should have reasonable time limits for their completion and should be measurable, specific, and attainable.

Another management function associated with setting objectives is *planning and control*. Planning is a specification of the means necessary to attain the goals set. Defining the method to achieve the goals establishes specific limits that can be used as standards for control. The manager carefully follows the specified means chosen, and the plan will automatically meet the standards set. Control of this function is thereby insured. Since plans are derived from objectives, they become a means for attaining objectives. However, plans should be flexible so that the organization can adapt quickly to new situations, especially in the areas of personnel planning, capital expenditure, operational expenditure, and space requirements. Thus planning creates criteria and standards of action and behavior for that department, and these again become the basis for control. Control also involves the necessity for knowing what is going on. If he is properly established, the manager will know what standards are being met, what objectives have been attained, and what changes are necessary to maintain momentum.

To serve as guides for the department members, *policies* need to evolve from planning; in effect, they establish precedent and specify responses to events. Since all members of the department are guided by the same policies, their behavior becomes predictable and stability within the department is insured. Finally, since clear policies provide a framework for individual decisions, they may encourage *delegation* of decision making in specific circumstances. That the policies be respected by the director is obviously important.

Since every organization consists of human beings who are vital to the department's performance, another important function of the manager is to *recruit, select,* and *develop* the human resources. Finally, he must *integrate* the personnel into the effort toward attaining the hospital's overall goals. To do so, he must be able to *communicate* effectively; for if he cannot transmit his ideas to others, his work may be wasted no matter how sound his objectives and how well thought out his planning. People in the organization have a need for information at all levels, and they do seek it. Their need for information should be met by establishing communication on a two-way basis, since each component of a department must have the information needed to operate efficiently.

The last of the manager's functions is to *supervise* and *motivate* his subordinates. That process involves day-to-day supervision of personnel who are assigned tasks by the manager or his delegate. It should be noted that the management process as described here is a cyclic recurring pattern that is modified as necessary.

There is at present no significant literature on management for the physician, but there is an extensive literature on hospital administration, health care, and the business sphere. The plethora of texts may be confusing, but the essentials of the management process are the same no matter what the environment; thus nonmedical sources may be of use.[6,7] Inferences can be made from these other studies because of common structural similarities and implicit operational principles.

THE ESSENTIAL ELEMENTS OF
SUCCESSFUL MANAGEMENT

Since formal data were difficult to obtain in the medical field, a study in depth of a different field must be used to illustrate the problems of successful management. The U.S. Small

Business Administration conducted an extensive study of the life history of 194 varied small businesses totally unrelated to medicine.[8] The complexity and scope of these operations and their problems were, however, strikingly similar to those observed in the limited medical study previously referred to. The common denominator of the two groups was total absence of prior management training. Fifty percent of businesses failed within five years. The underlying causes of the failures were limited to a small number of recurring deficiencies that were not observed in the businesses that were labeled successful because they were financially solvent and operating after more than five years. The factors were weighted by their frequency of occurrence and their estimated importance as causes of failure. They are

1. Drive, with a relative weight of 3 in 9
2. Thinking ability, with a relative weight of 2 in 9
3. Communication ability, with a relative weight of 2 in 9
4. Human relations ability, with a relative weight of 1 in 9
5. Technical ability, with a relative weight of 1 in 9

Drive. The single most important ingredient of success was drive, which is subdivided into responsibility, vigor, initiative, persistence, and health. All are obvious and self-explanatory, but some further elaboration of their application to the medical field may be useful. Responsibility implies *relevance*, which was a problem with medical directors. The directors who had trouble had a misdirected drive to goals other than those the institution had selected. If you are to be the "hospital's man," you obviously must adopt the hospital's long-term goals and plan.

For the same reason, misdirection in vigor and persistence are also somewhat detrimental. Directors failed to demonstrate adequate responsibility for and dedication to the objectives—or in some instances refused to acknowledge the objectives—of the departments they were to manage. They could not sacrifice any personal plan or needs for the good of the department, and they were rather superficial when they attempted to meet the dedicatory need. Since the medical director was an independent contractor, he was free to allocate his time to various departmental tasks depending upon his evaluation of the problems. It was obvious, however, that in many instances he either did not delegate enough time to meet the specific situation or did not devote enough effort to developing a new approach that would satisfy the requirements within the time limit established.

Thinking ability. The components of this essential are original, critical, creative, and analytical thinking. The medical director, if he is to be leader, must be able to demonstrate effectively, to those who sit in judgment upon his performance, that he has the capacity to guide the department intelligently rather than merely react to each new problem. A common fault noted in the medical survey was the lack of preventive action and planning. Some problems were handled appropriately; others were not; and, amazingly, still others were merely explained away. This behavior aberration sooner or later came to the notice of someone at a higher level of authority. If the director had been performing the required thinking function, he would have been able to anticipate a number of these problems before they reached a critical level. With repetitive crisis it became obvious to others that he was not responding appropriately, and failure of management was noted.

Communication ability. Somehow, in dealing with his staff, the director equated his ascendant position with the right to monopolize all the speaking time. He thus demonstrated failure to understand the process of communication, which consists of (1) listening and verbal comprehension (what is the other person trying to say?) and (2) oral and written communication (can the director get his message through to the listeners?). This was a frequent defect, particularly among the most articulate, since their monopoly of the verbalizing process in effect blocked input from those in subservient positions. The result was that a solution chosen was based upon incomplete data. That, of course, violates one of the prime managerial directives: the necessity to have enough input that planning and control are relevant. Additionally, although verbally articulate, the directors failed to make adequate written reports that busy administrators require for their planning and control.

Human relations ability. Components of this trait are ascendancy (feeling and acting as a leader), emotional stability (refraining from indulging one's own emotion at the expense of another), sociability (ability to relate to others appropriately and establish a close working contact with everyone), and cautiousness (not overreacting either in a personal or business relationship). Although there was no shortage of the first trait, ascendancy, there were relative deficiencies in the others, particularly in the related trait of consideration. Obviously, if he is to lead, the director must be able to see enough of the other person's point of view to take it into consideration. Most physicians were unable to consider the perception of the problem by a nonphysician; therefore, much of their communication and empathic efforts were wasted.

Another primary requirement in occupations with a considerable stress level is cheerfulness, since it is commonly associated with a positive attitude. If the leader has a positive attitude, he may be able to transmit it to the others and obtain the augmented group response he needs. Cooperation and tactfulness are equally important, since the director and his department are, after all, only components of a larger hospital team. Failure to integrate your specific activity into the overall purpose of the institution not only is personally annoying to others at your own peer levels but may be disruptive to the whole hospital's efforts in patient care.

Technical ability. To even be considered as a medical director, one must obviously have the additional training, expertise, and understanding of the specific techniques, tools, activities, and problems of the department he is to direct. The formal screening process required for medical staff membership is the only presently existing criterion. I am not aware of any instances in which a director "moved" purely because of lack of technical competence. However, if he is to manage rather than act as a technical consultant, he should have minimal reservations about using others' talents and abilities to supplement or complement his own.

THE HAZARDS OF DELEGATION

For effective departmental function, managerial time is essential. Thus you will find it necessary to delegate, both at the medical and at the technical levels. At whatever level, you must make a specific assumption regarding the competency of the person to whom you have subcontracted that task. To provide the adequate control, you must stipulate limits and guidelines so that lower-level decision making can be coordinated with total departmental function. Obviously, the lower the level the narrower the degrees of freedom you allow the person subcontracted for the task. Additionally, for effective delegation, you establish a clear definition of the specific responsibilities and authority limits attached to that particular function. The employee you have chosen should be capable of doing more than his position requires, but you must have some way you can check up on outcome to see how well he is exercising his independence of action. The performance criteria should be based on objective goals rather than on means.

Although delegation, as a managerial activity, has many problems, there is one problem that is unique to medicine. It is a consequence of excessive delegation in a particular field of activity. As a physician, your peers expect you to act the part and "do the doctoring" as well as whatever bureaucratic paperwork is necessary. When your managerial and administrative tasks grow so onerous and critical that you, to free up the time you need, may be tempted to delegate all of the medical activities to your associates, pause and think again. That could lead to a "palace revolution" unless you are so ego-dominant no one would dare challenge you as a leader. Otherwise, you should maintain your singular ability to perform effectively as a doctor to keep your associates in line.

This is the old struggle between the line and staff officers in the military and in business. The less experienced and less mature see only one criterion of superiority, namely, the medical technical ability that they possess. Thus the medical director's burden is that he must be able to do both tasks even though, from a viewpoint of efficiency, concentrating upon the general areas would be more productive in the long term.

THE ROLE OF PERSONAL PHILOSOPHY

In medicine, personal philosophy is perhaps the area of greatest divergence between managers who are physicians and those who are not. In the health care field, the nonphysician hospital managers realistically have no independent existence; professionally speaking, they are only parts of larger organizations. Therefore, under the behavioral and conditioning pressures exerted, they gradually adopt the philosophy and the goals of the organizations with which they are affiliated. Consequently, little attention has been paid to the individual's personal philosophy, since for long-term success it must blend well with the organizational philosophy.

The reverse is true in medicine. During his formative years, the physician is trained to think of himself as a unique individual both in medical school and in his specialty training. His activities and involvement in any team are peripheral, and he is denied the advantage of any formal training in how to blend with a concerted effort. Add to that the doctor's unique legal posture: the almost exclusive right to practice medicine. So at the same organizational level as a manager in industry, he will have far more authority and powers and independence for an appointment of equivalent responsibility. Thus the doctor will have evolved a service philosophy that will be at some variance with that of the organization.

As human beings, physicians have no problem in responding appropriately to stimuli for which they have been previously and appropriately conditioned. However, when the physician is confronted with situations for which no previous program exists, it will be his philosophical basis that will likely determine the nature and extent of his reaction. Thus the physician, never having been programmed to work with a team, much less as leader of it, is likely to run into situations that will require a response from him for which he has no established guidelines.

The director must, if he is to fulfill the requirements of his position honestly, subject his own performance to the same searching scrutiny he directs upon other members of his department. If he has not done so previously, he must at this time decide whether he can label himself a natural leader or whether he is essentially a loner. Certainly previous training and selection pressure may have contributed to that attribute; but even when he suspects a deficiency, he is capable of change with training in self-development.

If you are in fact interested in people, no matter what your personality type, you can mold your behavior patterns to make necessary human interaction tolerable and effective. If you are a "leadership-oriented person," you must work extensively upon your techniques of handling situations.

If you are a loner without desire to change, then you can make do by allowing another person to take over the functions informally so you retain the title and prerogatives of leader. Hospital administrators welcome the opportunity to assume the total leadership role via their department supervisors if the medical director abdicates. However, such choices should be made consciously so that you can watch for signs of trouble if different performance expectations arise. If no other model exists in the community, your performance may be accepted as reasonable by the department, administration, and medical staff.

A potential problem is that your legal assumption of the obligations of leadership is not lessened merely because you do not act like a leader. For example, if you subcontract all of the personnel surveillance function to your supervisor who is not particularly apt at recruitment, selection, and training, you may end up with incompetent personnel. You will be legally responsible if a serious problem should arise. So if you are to be a loner (technical consultant), a competent department supervisor is doubly essential.

PLANNING

Personal philosophy and character traits again will have a significant impact upon the type of planning activities the director is most likely to choose. In this regard the following quotation has particular relevance to medical planning.[9]

> Regardless of the organization concerned (business, government, military) the first and most significant problem with planning operations is the tendency to think of detailed planning as the most critical stage of the planning process. This approach leads people to focus quickly on the superficially most attractive alternative courses of action so as to get on with the "real work" of detailed planning. Associated with this problem is the tendency for plan-

ners to see events and deadlines in the near future in an exaggerated perspective compared with those further off in time. Decision makers also have a strong disinclination to rethink basic assumptions, to reconsider abandoned alternatives, or consider previously ignored alternatives once they have invested a substantial amount of time and effort in planning and promoting one course of action. When planning is done in a group, the problem is magnified. Staff members are inclined to follow the group consensus rather than rethink the logic that leads to the leader's decisions.

Essentially, acute medicine is a short-term activity; only in preventive medicine do we give thought to long-range consequences. The director must, in determining the departmental future goals, actively counter his tendency to hop from one short-term goal to another in favor of a long-range approach. The starting point should be an analysis of the department's function in terms of the hospital's long-range needs. The medical director should also list his own professional long-range objectives. Hopefully the two lists are not on divergent courses.

Having listed and identified the goals of the department and hospital, the director should interpret them for their individual impact upon the current departmental operation and function. The next step is to consider innovation and search for new opportunities. Planners should, rather than rely totally on fixed thinking and past events, search for new methods, products, and services that fit into the situation. Given the accelerating technological changes, the problem will be to pick out the appropriate changes from a host of many. Determining the impact of those probabilities upon your department and hospital will require many factual data that may not be easy to obtain. You should transmit such data as are available to the primary physicians and let them speculate and vocalize on their felt future needs. The final steps involve writing out a long-term plan of action that may include such items as budget revisions and capital equipment requests, new personnel policies, and training procedures.

To restate the planning process in a more formal fashion, the medical director, to exercise his authority, must act as a decision maker. He must be aware that even taking no action at all in response to events is a decision. He should also know that if he does not respond to the pressure of change, someone else certainly will. Elements in this *decision process* are:

1. Obtaining information as to change in status, at any level, of both department and hospital.
2. Analyzing the data for their significant impacts upon current departmental performance.
3. Measuring, if possible, department performance changes under the new circumstances.
4. Building a model of projected responses in terms of long-range goals.
5. Evolving the strategies to initiate the reactive changes and testing them for relevance.
6. Checking the new performance against predicted outcome based upon the model.

The medical director should try to avoid the temptation to respond only to short-term problems and ignore long-term trends. To that end he must establish a continuing dialogue with his associates and the members of the hospital staffs with whom he interacts on a regular basis so he can improve his perspective with different levels of input.

LEADERSHIP

Since leadership is one of the essential dimensions of management, we need to elaborate in some detail how it relates to management theory. All forms of leadership entail the exercise of authority in order to achieve the aims of the group (or its leader). According to McGregor,[10] there are two pure models of leadership with a wide continuum of mix in between. The two opposite positions are Theory X, which assumes that man is motivated by fear and basic needs (money), and Theory Y, which assumes that man is motivated by self-esteem and needs for self-actualization. Thus the Theory X managers create work environments that are highly centralized and highly structured; their concern is the external control of employees' work. Theory X management is characterized by close supervision and financial incentives. Theory Y managers create work environments that are decentralized and involve participative management by key employees. Self-direction results in self-growth and the creation of a humanistic organization rather than a bureaucratic or traditional organization. This approach, however, requires much more intensive work-up of each individual to determine his capabilities for independent action; for the leader is still the leader and is responsible for the results.

Both Theory X and Theory Y rely heavily upon mechanisms involved in the concept of the *self-fulfilling prophecy*. If in actual practice you label someone as an XYZ and then continue treating him as an XYZ, eventually he will begin to act like an XYZ because he believes he is an XYZ. A more destructive variant of this mechanism, when used for emotional or discriminatory reasons, is the *variable level of expectations*. Operationally these leader and supervisory personnel have difficulty treating all employees on an equal scale. That is manifested by (1) denying the existence of the mechanism and by (2) setting the criterion of adequate performance at different levels for different individuals. Thus certain individuals will find that they can never meet the standards expected of them no matter what their performance, and others (who may be even less competent, as, for example, in cases of nepotism) may easily match the requirements set for them.

Depending upon the social and personal factors present, that can be a morale-destroying operation. Thus it might be argued that all the criteria of adequate performance should be generated logically and objectively and should be common knowledge. But neither a Theory X nor a Theory Y manager would condone such a policy. You may actually find Theory X and Theory Y leadership behavior in the same department applied to different people at the same time or to the same people at different times.

Hopefully, the best leader will use as much of Theories X and Y as the situation calls for but more specifically will demonstrate the type of direction and support that is operationally necessary at the moment. To those of the staff who need specific direction he will and must provide it, whereas at the same time he will allow

others to run on a loose rein. The ratio of the two components X
and Y will vary from hour to hour and from day to day and from
situation to situation. If the medical director and his supervisor are
doing their job properly, they will start each new employee off in a
Theory X control situation. Then, by the use of consistent review
of the individual's actual and potential abilities coupled with relevant in-service training, they will ultimately transform him into an
individual who can be controlled by Theory Y management.

Some departments are so large and have been in operation so
long that the hospital has taken over leadership of both personnel
and operation except for the strictly medical members and
functions of the department. That is most particularly true of
Pathology, Anesthesiology, and Radiology. There the medical director can exercise leadership only by interacting positively with
key management personnel who, by time-honored custom, "run
the department." Since the director is still legally responsible for
the actions of those personnel, he needs to be certain that the
supervisor will exercise the control that he no longer has. So although he may not be directly involved in specific leadership activity, he had best be certain that the leadership activity exerted in his
behalf is something that he can live with.

On the other hand, in new clinical departments where there is
no supply or heritage of middle management talent the director
may have to exercise a far greater degree of leadership until the lack
of adequate and appropriate training of the assigned staff can be
corrected—at least at the supervisory level. In this situation he will
have to dedicate time not only to observe and review but also to sit
and counsel people about their problems and their hang-ups. And
although that time will be well spent, he will unfortunately be at
the mercy of criticism from his peers about what they assume to be
fraternization rather than personnel management and leadership.

RECRUITING

Recruiting is another attribute that is a spin-off of
leadership: you must have the ability to attract people of compe-

tence to your department. In an exponentially expanding field the ability to obtain an adequate supply of competent talent is extremely valuable, particularly in those specialties in which formal training requirements have not yet been established and no large pool of talent is available.

In addition, recruiting is part of management; for you must do *manpower planning*—you must predict the growing needs of the department, present and future, and the changing characteristics of the personnel required. Manpower planning begins with manpower inventories, which include reviews of available talent and the skills for positions available; estimations of the loss expected through attrition, layoffs, promotions, transfers, and dismissals; and study of the current departmental employees to see if they are adequate for current and immediate needs. If the review turns up significant deficiencies, can the deficiencies be corrected by upgrading and in-service training or must you obtain new talent? Finally, you must formally forecast the department's future needs for different kinds of skills and experience so that you can begin the search process.

Personnel function does have another management aspect that is of immense initial importance to the new director. What is the hospital's personnel philosophy, and what is the personnel strategy of the new department? Will the approach be to hire the best class of talent available no matter the cost, or will it be to hire minimally competent people who just meet legal and employment requirements? If the latter, will you then be expected to upgrade those minimally competent people to the necessary level with on-the-job training and in-service programs?

PRECEDENT SETTING

When you settle in as leader of the department, everyone will observe you closely to see how you react to each situation; for each new response establishes a precedent. Being aware of that, and since operationally you need that consistency, you should carefully reflect before arriving at a decision on how to respond. Your staff will expect you to use that same response in that same situation from then on. Consistent behavior of leaders gives subordinates increased freedom, since they are able to predict the leader's behavior. Thus you might say that *consistency is the mother of credibility*; for your staff will be able to rely on your behavior and provide the support that the situation calls for. The leader's problem here is that the situation may not be exactly similar to an earlier one and so a different response is called for. If he responds differently, the director is obligated to explain why; otherwise, consternation and confusion may ensue. This is particularly important when corrective action is required.

Personnel of traditional departments must conform to set educational patterns and often obtain licenses. Consequently, they have assurance as to their individual worth: it is documented. On the contrary, staff members of newer departments potentially suffer from a sense of inferiority and frustration: their acceptance is entirely predicated upon leader and group approval, which often is quite variable. Such people, who are unsure of themselves, do not respond well to abrupt challenges to their status, since that is merely based on on-the-job training (a variable experience), ambivalent emotion, and their ego. Consequently, when errors that require correction occur, abrasive types of reprimand are particularly likely to be disastrous to their self-esteem. Since they are entitled to the benefits of "due process," the director should first investigate the source of the deficiency. Was it due entirely to the personnel error, somebody else's error, improper on-the-job or in-service training, inadequate equipment, ambiguous or incorrect orders, or some extraordinary situation?

Unwise and frequent criticism, particularly if delivered in public, will quickly erode and destroy individual performance and perhaps even the spirit of the entire group if the action is unwarranted. Certainly, unless well deserved, the members of the group can foresee the same thing happening to them, and since they can not be certain that it will never happen to them, they will respond appropriately. Thus one can get a whole department acting in a defensive manner that may be disastrous in terms of departmental efficiency. The director has to establish credibility that any judgment will be adequately researched and fair, that the appropriate action will be taken in a manner to retain the technicians' self-respect, and that the supervisor's performance will be the same under the same types of stress.

Both director and supervisor must insure that each error accountable to the department is investigated and handled at an appropriate level and is not merely passed downstream to staff in a pecking-order assignment of fault. Spontaneous and unwise reprimands in public are an indirect insult and should be forbidden in the policy manual. The offended person may be so upset that he begins seeking a position elsewhere. The persons most likely to commit open errors in the department are those who are the most motivated activists. In general, the least well trained, who are aware of their deficiency, will rarely place themselves in such an exposed position.

MOTIVATION

Maslow,[11] in his study of motivation, identified five levels from which drive originates. They range from the most basic (security and food) to the most intellectual (developing one's self-identity). Today anyone can easily satisfy basic needs on welfare. Therefore, people working under nonideal circumstances, such as those of hospitals, must be motivated by some other benefits than the salary that buys the food and lodging. Both Theory X and Theory Y imply the presence of other factors as a source of purposeful behavior. The other benefits are not restricted to sickness, vacation, and retirement benefits but more importantly include a sense of identity, treatment as a human being, and recognition of individual worth and capability, all of which culminate in acceptance by and the respect of their peer group and their leader. The higher benefits can best be attained by the director interacting with the person on a one-to-one basis in a positive situation. However, all too often the staff's only intimate personal contact with the medical director is in short-lived disciplinary situations. That is not positive conditioning.

The time to begin providing the nonfiscal benefits is at the be-

ginning of employment. The break-in period is of particular importance in hospital departments with complex tasks and large staffs;
for it is then that the director and supervisor can most effectively
establish a positive behavior pattern in the mind of the new employee. People who have just been hired are likely to be in a state
of increased receptivity to demand for their skills and talents. If the
director and supervisor totally ignore the recruit and turn him over
to a rote type of orientation program, the recruit may then decide
that this is not the time and place to open up and do his or her best.

Such decisions are not made consciously; they are triggered by
the unconscious effect of the total Gestalt of the new work situation. Thus the director must be involved in the screening and selection process, in the orientation program, and in the continuing
educational program if he is to provide the high-grade rewards that
many seek. It is essential that the medical director build up rapport
with his employees not only so he can reward them but also so
they can mutually support each other in doing the department's
work more adequately and in becoming an information resource. In
very large departments such an approach may be practical on a
long-term basis only by concentrating on the new recruits.

SYSTEMS ANALYSIS OF QUALITY OF CARE

Operationally, hospitals are such complex functions
encompassing services, processes, geographical units, and product
activities that only a systems analysis approach will permit dissec-
tion of the entire chain of circumstances that is involved in the
delivery of a particular health service. Systems analysis recognizes
that all parts are so interrelated and interdependent as to form the
whole, and it is a study of those interrelations and interdependen-
cies. One variable interacting with another variable results in a
gradual chain reaction throughout the whole system. Systems
analysis is of the highest priority for those departments with a 24-
hour-day, 7-day-week operation. The reason is that surveillance
and supervision over the entire 168 hours a week is less likely to be
uniformally adequate, so the systems analysis must extend over

time as well as over geography. Deficiencies or weak links must be identified before they can be corrected. Characteristically, the problems are the interaction points between various departments that are involved in providing the total care package. The following is a systems analysis of the chain of care required for patient benefit in a therapeutic service. Each separate element must be examined for (1) completeness and (2) proper integration with its contiguous elements:

1. The actual medical condition (need) of that patient in that hospital.
2. The ability of the patient's physician to identify the treatable aspects of the patient's condition and develop a rational treatment plan.
3. The physician's pertinent and chronologically appropriate orders based upon a rational treatment plan.
4. The transcription of the physician's orders to appropriate forms and transmission of those orders or forms to the appropriate departments without error.
5. Receipt of the order by the appropriate department and initiation of the steps to put it into effect without undue delay. That entails comprehension of the intent of the order.
6. Availability of the equipment appropriate to the needed service.
7. Availability of the staff with sufficient training and enough time to adequately perform the service requested.
8. The degree of cooperation of other departments interacting with the patient at the time the service is to be provided, including patient availability.
9. The degree of patient cooperation with the performance of the service because he understands what is happening, that is, he is adequately prepared for services to satisfy his needs.
10. The efficacy and accuracy of delivery of service or product.
11. Abstraction of objective data about the results of service on that patient.
12. The feedback to the physician of the results (data) of the

service so that the physician may modify his original treatment plan as necessary.

Systems analysis in medicine has been developed under the title of Problem-Oriented Medical Records, a nationwide activity stemming from the efforts of Dr. Lawrence L. Weed.[12] Medical audit systems will also focus on the complex chains of delivery of health care when simpler problems have been handled. Thus before any corrective or disciplinary action is to be taken, the site and level of the failure of service must first be identified. One problem that has had too little attention is the development of criteria for determining the success of product delivery.

Another significant factor in the analysis of chains of care is the degree to which the patient's physician defers judgmental decisions regarding therapy to personnel delivering the therapy. Although such deference is appropriate at some level of care and feasible if adequate resources exist, as, for example, the intensive or coronary care nurse, in other circumstances it may represent gross misapplication of the concept. Here the problem is that the physician is not putting enough of his own time and attention into acquiring the background necessary to make his own decisions.

Another systems problem is the presence of adequate numbers of staff with sufficient training, appropriate equipment, and enough time to render the therapy services ordered. That is one of the most pressing concerns of the director; on paper the department may be adequately serviced, but in actual practice the available services may be entirely sporadic. The folk saying "out of sight, out of mind" exemplifies the nonsystems approach to staffing a department that is operational for most of the 168 hours per week. If the medical director and supervisor characteristically work the prime time (Monday to Friday, 9:00 to 5:00), then the personnel on that shift, if both leaders are conscientious, will be very well trained indeed. However, the non-prime-hours staff will have to operate independently—without the backup of director and supervisor—yet will encounter as wide an array of serious problems as those seen in the daylight hours. Because of their isolation from the source of training, upgrading, and enriching, they may not be able to cope and indeed may perform inadequately. The automatic response will be disciplinary action, not more supportive attention, even though that would be the logical solution.

TABLES OF ORGANIZATION

If you are taking over an already established position, then you may have to deduce exactly how the lines of authority are set up in that particular department before attempting any changes. But if the department is a new one, you may wish to suggest a particular table of organization that is in keeping with your specialty and your management philosophy. The three basic patterns are graphically displayed in the figure on the next page. In the first type, A, the director is in a cul-de-sac and his input is very limited, so he is essentially a technical adviser/consultant. Because he is out of the mainstream of communication, he can easily be bypassed and thus is likely to be ineffective in exercising control apart from activities that are specifically his responsibility. If he is labeled medical director in the contract, then he is at the mercy of the supervisor who is acting in his stead, since he will be operationally unaware of the business of the department.

The second model, B, is a hybrid. The medical director has direct responsibilities and control over aspects of departmental activity and answers to the administrator. But the supervisor has the same channels; and if he is there more than the director, then obviously his control and input will predominate. Although model B is an improvement over model A, the director can still easily be bypassed if any points at issue come up. Theoretically, the director can also bypass the supervisor, but that is really not feasible unless he is prepared to spend as much time and effort in the department as the supervisor. In the absence of active opposition and with the connivance of administration and supervisor, model B can be converted to model A by gradually withdrawing information and access to control from the medical director.

The third type, C, is a chain of command that puts the director at the hub of communication and responsibility and is most in

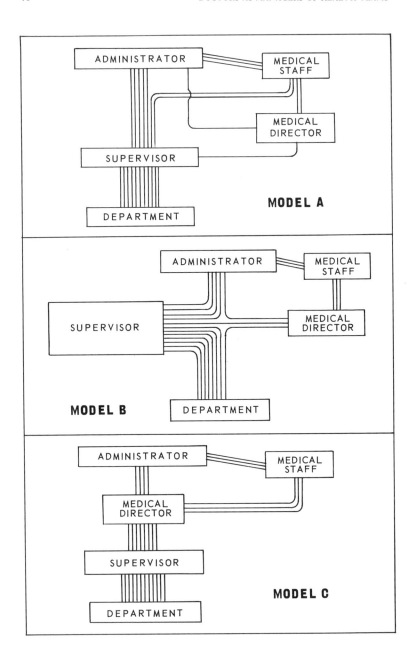

keeping with the recommendations of the Joint Commission on Accreditation of Hospitals. All communication, with the exception of routine minutiae of departmental business, goes through the director on its way to administration and the reverse. The director may waive the necessity for seeing certain regular reports on a weekly or monthly basis, but he has operational access to all information. Should the supervisor try to slip information around him, and he learns of the information from other sources, he should immediately investigate to prevent any buildup by a bypass. Obviously, C is the most administratively responsible model, but as a consequence it requires a considerably greater time commitment than either model A or model B. If you can provide only minimal departmental time, avoid model C; otherwise, you will wind up defeating your purpose. I would recommend David Starkweather's study[13] for the reader who wishes to pursue this matter in greater detail.

To whom is the director responsible? In answer, most hospital administrators tend to invoke the golden rule: "He who pays the gold, rules." According to it, the administrator obviously is in direct control of the medical director. However, in all of the tables of organization the medical staff also have input both directly and indirectly, so the medical director is also answerable to them professionally although not fiscally. One must also consider the fact that the administrator is a delegated agent of the Board of Trustees of the hospital, and so the medical director, like every other member of the hospital staff, ultimately answers to the Board. In an operational and functional sense, however, the buck stops at the administrator's desk.

In the event of a major policy difference as a result of which administrator and director disagree over the approach to be used, the director should remember that the Board of Trustees is available as the final arbitrator. Theoretically, everyone in the institution from the Board down responds to the philosophy of service of the institution. Now, the dispute may involve the interpretation of that philosophy, but the director must realize that the administrator will have a major voice in any interpretation.

THE SOURCE AND RESOLUTION OF CONFLICTS

Hospitals, except those whose medical staffs are entirely on salary, are organizationally unique in complexity of management authority, whence the potential for serious conflict. The most notable reason for complexity is the dual power base: the hospital's organizational structure with its administrator operating in tandem with the cohesively massive power of the independent medical staff. There are checks and balances to keep this union viable. The hospital's organizational structure is much more cohesive, efficient, and powerful and has tremendous resources in personnel and finances, *but* it is totally dependent upon the physicians' patronage. In organizational function and strength the medical staff structure is as a David to the hospital's Goliath, *but* the ability to shift patients elsewhere can reduce the administrator's power toward zero as his hospital empties.

However, it is the physicians' overpowering independence that is the prime source of their weakness. They cannot pull together for long unless their own personal interests are involved. Thus the administrator is driven to seeking a constituency from among the medical staff to obtain long-term security, and the price is that he must share with the medical staff some of his monolithic powers. So the pair of one-legged dancers continue in their halting minuet. There is a basic difference in perspective between the administration who must look at both the short-term costs and the long-term trends and the physician who sees only the patient he is treating with a viewpoint that may be very short-term indeed. When you mix into decision-making levels the administrators and the equally strong-willed physicians, you may have significant differences of opinion. Schulz and Johnson[14] have discussed in detail this one aspect of hospital administration.

Thus, at some point in time, almost every medical director is drawn into a position of significant disagreement with the administration. The disagreement may remain totally aboveboard and be resolved in a logical fashion by majority opinion. The medical director should realize that the administrators, if they choose, can so erode his position that their opinion carries the day even in public forum. Since the administrators have a deeper and more sophisticated appreciation of management function and politics than the doctors, their first line of attack is to isolate the director by cutting off his information sources and thus his input. The next step involves reducing his operating control under the tables of organization. That type of undercutting of lines of authority requires the full cooperation of the departmental supervisor.

If for whatever reason the supervisor will not cooperate, the administrator may be blocked in that approach. If he is, he then can harass the department by attacking its nonessential operations by delays in budget, staff appropriations, and so on. He can take the matter to the Executive Committee, if he feels that the issue is serious enough to warrant an open challenge, and from there to the Board of Trustees. His ultimate weapon is to cancel the contract. But that step requires a legally valid reason, and, often because of the medical director's own political strength and power base, he is usually reluctant to take it. What he can do is to wait for the contract to expire and then refuse to renew it until the issues can be resolved to his satisfaction. Of course, if the director has had the forethought to include an automatic renewal clause in his contract, that ploy cannot be used.

When under administrative fire, the medical director has several methods of defense depending upon his understanding of management process and his own awareness of the situation. He can respond to the cutting of communication by developing other channels to keep him informed. Those channels must be independent of the regular lines of authority in the hospital; but if they are based upon reliable sources, they are just as valuable. If the supervisor is "on the doctors' side" and pressures are exerted upon the other operational functions of the department, the director can respond by barraging administration with written memoranda requesting all of the activities that suddenly are delayed and pointing out that this has never occurred before. He should avoid two defense measures that the unsophisticated tend to use immediately: (1) raising the boogeyman of impaired patient care unless that is really happening and (2) being a roadblock to communication from the medical staff, since that may adversely affect patient care.

If the conflict over the issues continues, the next step should be to write up detailed position papers about the matter under dispute and send copies to administration and the medical staff through the appropriate committee structures. The strategy is to keep the matter out in the open where the rules are different but in the director's favor. Normally a director does not submit much written material to committees except on request and as a year-end report. A director's written reports therefore become a defense tactic that is very effective provided his position is correct and aboveboard. The reports should be very well written out and should utilize the superior background, experience, and training of the director to point out better alternatives than those proposed by the opposing camp. Remember, even if the alternatives are superior, they can still be defeated in open committee unless they are adequately buttressed with wide support.

A fourth background defense is to intensify the public relations activities with the medical staff and other key hospital employees who have influence. This will be difficult to do unless the director already is interacting with regularity. If he is beset by both administration and his own supervisor, he can also utilize the "informal leaders" referred to in Chapter 3 as potential allies in the department to keep tabs on events and continue some managing input even from the sidelines.

If the key figure in the conflict is the supervisor, who sides with the administrator and may even have recommended the measures you are opposing, you may be able, by sheer guts, determination, and staying power, to wear the supervisor down to the point where either he vacates the position or capitulates and agrees to work with you. That, of course, strains all departmental relationships, but at least you have demonstrated that you can use your power adequately and your opinion cannot be ignored. All this, of course, is predicated upon your being reasonably correct in your own stand and prepared to make compromises if necessary.

However, if serious conflicts should arise and the director comes through successfully, he must be aware he may be living on borrowed time from that moment on. Few administrators can appreciate being frustrated at their own game; fewer still can forgive and forget.

COMMUNICATION AND FEEDBACK

The supervisor has a responsibility to determine exactly what his department is doing in the hospital, and from that he will generate current status reports. In addition to keeping administration informed, the reports enable him to react to any new situation. The medical director must have that information, but in addition he must seek information from a wider area—the department's integration with the hospital's effort. The supervisor has his daily, weekly, and monthly reports and the advantage of attending the weekly hospital management council. He should pass that information on to the medical director as a matter of routine. The medical director, however, cannot rely upon his supervisor as the only source of information; he must also develop multiple parallel sources of information to be certain that what he is hearing is substantially correct rather than slanted. With only a single source he can easily become a captive and a pawn of the source with all the potential complications.

The major principle the director must be aware of is that *needed information never volunteers itself.* If the director merely sits in his office with a sign on the door saying "The Boss: Welcome; Come In," he will rarely hear a complete story of anything. In this regard he must emulate the wardheelers of the Eastern cities in the early 1900s. Those gentlemen traveled up and down their precincts stopping to say, "Hello, how are you?" By talking to people and by going through a variety of ritualistic social contact patterns, they received much valuable information, both current and background. All of that information was volunteered spontaneously, and presumably most of it might never have been reported via official channels. The problem with information is that no one but you can evaluate its importance to you. Therefore, you have to hear it to evaluate it; no one can screen for you. You may thus receive a very large amount of data that serve no purpose but to give you a better background, but you must maintain your practice of open input to get the crucial facts you need.

The director must thus display traits of sociability including the capacity to dedicate time to listening without indicating he is in a hurry and without trying to dominate the conversation. His attention and concern for others, both in and out of his department, will undoubtedly bring forth much information, only a small portion of which may be useful to him. Those sources are, however, invaluable only if he continues to cultivate them, since they in effect are independently corroborative sources of the workings of his department and the hospital as a whole.

The director must be aware of the tremendous importance of body language, that is, how to express his availability or nonavailability to hospital personnel who need his time and attention. Will he listen to them with respect and circumspection, or will he snap off their heads because they are bothering him? The information-gathering function may be viewed by his peers as unnecessary fraternization with the lower echelon, but it is nevertheless essential to management of the department and more particularly to the director's own survival.

Effective communication does not just happen. It requires the application of management functions to the structure, technology, and human factors of the hospital. Psychologists have studied communication networks in groups and have evaluated the transmission speed and the effectiveness on group members. Yet despite all the theory, hospitals are rapidly becoming a wasteland in terms of effective communication because of the block imposed by excessive amounts of data from multiple sources without corresponding improvement in data-handling capability.

At the turn of the century there were only two components of the health team, nurse and physician. The physician wrote in his particular section (progress notes) and read what the nurse wrote in hers (nurse's notes), and vice versa. The official channel of communication and command was the doctor's order sheet. Close control existed, since there was an adequate, easily negotiated channel of communication in both directions.

With the explosive growth of health services and sciences in the last three-quarters century, however, there are probably more than ten places on current hospital charts where vital information can be recorded daily. If the physician does not follow a systematic daily search pattern of each area of current department interaction with his patient, he may miss some vital information with a time fuse.

At the same time that we have the growth of specialized services we also have the removal of the nurse (and her key communication position) from the scene owing to economic pressures. With the nurse-to-patient ratio dropping, the nurse is no longer the effective coordinator of patient information that she formerly was. Consequently, much information, apart from laboratory and diagnostic studies, is now also transmitted by word of mouth with the built-in deficiencies of such an informal system.

Now, after this three-quarter century of progress, the ultimate in patient care is the special care unit. There again we have almost a one-to-one nurse-to-patient ratio, and so the nurse is again the key to the channel of patient information. However, the price of special care is considerably greater than that of standard care, and so it is restricted to problems deserving that cost. What this points out in terms of communication theory is that, to be effective, you need to speak to a source and the source has to be highly reliable, particularly in a rapidly changing situation.

Thus no matter what the department, the director also has a group of people who are in daily contact with some of the patients and from whom he can receive input with a minimum number of intermediary steps. There are any number of models of communication networks,[15] but the only model that is important to the director is one that he can construct on the basis of his access to people with data to report.

COMMUNITY STANDARDS AND COMMUNITY NEEDS

From the management point of view the director must determine what his peers are doing at the other hospitals in the community. This is not a case of looking for faults so one can display his superiority; it is a matter of learning what variety of working approaches are in current use. The trend was initiated by the fiscal intermediaries who are beginning to run comparisons between hospitals, and the approach is now on its way to becoming a standard practice. Compounding the problem are the mandatory quality control programs that are to be administered on a regional basis. Thus the unique personal types of approach to problems that have been so characteristic of U.S. medicine may be suddenly and rapidly challenged. The directors' only recourse is to band together in anticipation of such challenges and evolve a joint, regional approach in their particular specialties.

Unfortunately, the health profession is suffering from a rampant epidemic of the white hat–pure heart syndrome: the belief that merely because you wear a white hat (or a white coat), your heart is pure, and you possess a valid license to practice medicine, all your efforts are obviously relevant and useful and should be financially rewarding. There is a groundswell of a somewhat contrary view led by the federal government with its forthcoming quality control activity and augmented by a segment of the private sector with its increasing attention to malpractice issues. Thus it is becoming necessary to develop documentation that your department product is indeed relevant and beneficial. As expected, the attack is apparently being focused upon the newest clinical departments, those with the least patina of respectability, venerability, and tradition. Physician managers of clinical departments should be in the forefront of those establishing objective criteria that will enable scrutiny of departmental results with approval leading to speedy cost recovery for those services.

The problem is that this new task thrust primarily upon hospital-based physicians is unaccompanied by any additional public funds to accomplish its purpose. Thus it may be necessary to pool resources of many institutions to develop an approach that will satisfy all of the formal requirements. Obviously each medical director cannot fight his battle individually without additional funds being appropriated for that task. Managers, even though intrinsically competitive, will have to cooperate for this common purpose rather than vie for unique personal advantage over one another as is often the case today.

THE REWARDS OF MANAGEMENT

The preceding discussion may seem to indicate that management is an onerous grinding type of activity that requires not only a masochistic personality but also a willingness to give more of one's self than most honorable people would wish. That is not entirely correct. It is also a potentially rewarding and stimulating activity, but only if the director will allow himself to grow with the position. Under the stimulus of a continual barrage of problems, he may find an increase in maturity, wisdom, and experience at a rate and to a degree that he never would have encountered under less stringent circumstances. Not only will he reap professional benefits from his improved human relations and leadership skills but he can apply them to his own personal advantage. His necessary involvement and interaction with other departments will enrich his appreciation of just how to utilize the total health team resources for the benefit of the patients. Finally, his contact with decision-making levels of the hospital and his on-the-job training activities will enhance his psychological sensitivity in handling all grades of people and perhaps enable him to distinguish, with ever-increasing efficiency, the rough diamonds of talent in the multitudes whom he encounters each day.

MANAGEMENT ALTERNATIVES

Each director has a choice: operating independently as a technical adviser/consultant (but retaining the status and rewards of management) or assuming the mantle and responsibilities of manager and medical director. In both instances he should continue as a skilled specialist in his field. Under the first option the hospital will certainly substitute some fairly strong middle management person to operate the department with the director's occasional input. But there may be a downstream cost to this option. Under the second option the director, while not specifically remunerated for management activities, does obligate himself to guide the department effectively through its planned growth with ever-improving function. Economic downstream benefits are likely, but they depend upon his successful performance and the course of events.

Begin by listing the departmental problems, both current and future, and separate them into categories: those you will handle, those you will delegate, and those you will postpone. Establish a set of priorities for the problems that you will handle by determining, in concert with your coworkers and key department personnel, a solution in terms of short- and long-term objectives. Consider the relation between the various goals and make necessary adjustments. Propose an appropriate series of methods to attain those objectives with current resources. If the resources are insufficient, you generate a secondary level of objectives: acquiring the resources to meet the primary goals. At this point you must reevaluate the complex of goals and plans and develop an overall strategy to achieve them as effectively as possible.

I recommend that considerable attention and thought be devoted to trying to anticipate the nature and degree of any opposition and possible obstacles. Since the initially simple objectives have now developed into a long-term complex of activity, you will need to set guideposts that will serve to keep you on course; a prime essential (guidepost) is setting the *timing* and *sequence* of development and achievement. A very common stumbling block to implementation will be the acquisition of appropriate personnel as departmental activity expands. So the strategy must include personnel policies on upgrading, recruiting, and training with its own set of bench marks.

Department activity and expansion must then be monitored by many objective criteria to indicate trends. In the meantime, while acquiring as much help as you can on the way, you must continue integrating with and selling to the rest of the hospital teams the current product and the future goals of the department. Persist in efforts to develop a consensus (public relations), but be ready and willing to reexamine your situation and assist other departments in light of such new developments as advances in medical technology and demographic and social changes. With the new learning and maturity you have acquired in the process of developing the managerial approach you should regularly review the direction and implication of changes at all levels—personal, professional, and social—and make the appropriate course adjustments. At some time you will need to redirect your attention to the community and be prepared to cooperate on a regional basis in an effort to solve problems that are beyond the capabilities of individuals.

3

THE PERSONNEL FUNCTION

THE REAL LEADER

An opening exists and you have been chosen to fill it. You must explore in depth the job description, since it, and not your title, has bearing upon whether your leadership will be formal or informal. Frankly, will those in unquestioned authority delegate to you real powers of management, or will they use other channels to attain their ends? You may quickly establish your future position by defining the limits of your authority in the area of personnel management. In the best of all possible worlds you, as the formal (licensed) leader of the department whose theoretical authority is bounded only by the rules of the organization and prevailing law, are still advised to review the limits in a joint conference with the department supervisor and the administrator. For here you will find that, depending upon the nature of your affiliation, there are in extended discussion many reservations and qualifications with regard to department staff.

In the reverse situation, as an independent contractor, you may find that your formal influence upon the department staff is very indirect indeed. Thus in either case you will find that staff changes come very slowly unless you proceed to act in a rational, consistent, and reasonable manner. Then you may also assume the added influence of indirect authority, which, with your official position, takes the ball out of the supervisor's hands. To do so you must be aware of the facts of administrative life. Although legally as the named director you are responsible, the majority of administrators prefer to control these and other affairs, bypassing you with a person who is directly and totally responsible to them. So you will, therefore, find that most supervisors will do their best to maintain as much independence of you as possible in order not to compromise what they consider their primary loyalty.

Thus unless you are prepared to exert effective leadership, you may find yourself in an anomalous position wherein you are responsible for the professional conduct of the department staff yet have no voice in staff choice or control. To obtain the security of that influence will require significant personal involvement, acumen, and expertise in manipulating human relations. Porter, Lawler, and Hackman aptly summarize the problem of "how to" in the following quotation.[16]

> Management literature on leadership involves numerous theories and empirical findings and suggests that it is impossible to draw up perfect specifications for a leader. The major propositions of leadership studies indicate that:
>
> 1. Trait theory: There are a finite number of identifiable traits of effective leaders, and these traits, such as intelligence, ambition, self-confidence, etc., differentiate the effective from the ineffective leaders.
>
> 2. Situational theory: Effective leadership is determined by a combination of the characteristics of the leader such as personality, the requirements of the task, the followers' needs, attitudes, etc., and the organizational environment in which leaders and followers operate.
>
> 3. Behavioral theory I: The element of consideration—the effective leader is characterized by warm relationships with subordinates, uses general supervision rather than close supervision, is willing to explain his actions and willing to listen to subordinates, all without any implication of laxity or laissez faire behavior.
>
> 4. Behavioral theory II: Initiation of structures—the effective

leader is characterized by his performance in the initiating roles of planning, organizing, coordinating, directing, and controlling his subordinates' work activities.

The authors go on to say that to understand leadership is to view it as a process of influence which can be shared among members of a work group.

There are administrators who are without leadership capabilities; they cannot influence members of a group to accomplish desired goals. A director is a formal leader who can influence members of a group through resources that are at his disposal and are unavailable to other group members. These resources include control of information about tasks or environmental contingencies received from the hierarchy and the ability to reward with performance evaluation, bonuses, time off from work, and liberty to deviate from existing work practices. The leader has added influence through close association with legitimate authority in the management hierarchy. Lastly, he has expertise based on specialized knowledge that group members do not possess.

The leader can utilize his resources according to the situation and exert significant influence on the performance of the group. Porter et al. identified two major leadership functions: diagnosis and execution.[17]

Diagnosis must be made to determine what needs to be done to keep the group moving in the desired direction. It includes monitoring the environment for task demands and determining what kinds of member behaviors are critical to effective task performance. Execution involves taking specific action to deal with the needs of the group at the time, as revealed by the diagnosis. The leader must create conditions within the group that will increase motivation and interpersonal effectiveness, and take direct action through the utilization of sources of influence.

Unless you can seize the initiative and maintain momentum, you may find that your role is that of medical adviser/consultant to the department. Yet your title places upon you the obligation to get results even though you lack the influence to manage people and events to attain those results. So in these matters the first hurdle you will have to surmount is the idea that you must be perfect.

Though we all subscribe to the notion that no one is perfect, many of us nonetheless nurture the sneaking suspicion that we may be the rare exception, particularly on a situation-to-situation basis. If you act on that basis in human relations, you will insure that your career will be studded with a series of confrontations over minor matters of no moment; and that is likely to warp your development as a manager of people.

In the case in which you do admit to imperfection, you can study and listen and learn and experiment in the areas in which you recognize deficiency. In medicine we are aware of the shortcoming of basing long-term actions upon incomplete knowledge of the situation, and we are also aware that pat answers without further search for data are commonly equated with immaturity and lack of experience. Human relations are fully as complex as human diseases.

SITUATIONAL THINKING

As director you must proceed on the optimistic assumption that necessary skills will improve with enough time and dedication. In addition to the skills elaborated upon in Chapter 2, you must accent development of honesty of purpose, credibility, and empathy and the devotion of enough additional time to acquire the experience. A logical approach to a new area of endeavor is the assumption of an observational data-collecting mode as a learning device. Pigors and Myers call this "situational thinking." In order to understand and achieve a comprehensive picture of organizations and work, they consider three variables: the *human elements*, such as individual differences and interpersonal relations; the *technical factor*, which involves equipment and methods used in management procedures, methods used in production, wage and salary administration, and the like, and space-time dimensions and relations such as size and location of the working organization and office allocations and *organizational policy*, which becomes a factor in any situation in which it is interpreted and used as a guide.[18]

As the new leader you already know the technical aspects of

your specialty. Now you must study the employees for whom you are responsible. How do they perform the essential and integral department function? Indeed, how do they interact with other areas of hospital service? What impact do they have on the services you perform? Daily briefing sessions with the supervisor are essential until you have learned the rules and the positions of each player. This orientation time should be measured in days and weeks, not hours, if the department is at all complex.

RESISTANCE TO CHANGE

Resistance to change can and does occur at any and all levels. Miner addresses this point in the following statement:[19]

> All organizations experience continuous change. But people in organizations resist change, even though it has been a part of human experience as long as life itself. Whenever organizations experience change, it can happen in three different ways—through people, through structure, or through technology. Whenever people in organizations experience the impact of change, they resist it. The major reasons for this are: We have invested time and energy in things as they are presently functioning and change may endanger the equilibrium. Any change will create uncertainty unless that change brings with it some tangible benefits. In other words, "Resistance may stem from a threat to basic assumptions, personal values, sources of security, and friendship relationships."

The natural tendency, when challenged by the altered demands of and need for new skills in a different position, is to retreat to a performance area in which you are secure. That is a self-defeating mechanism for a director who is responsible for other personnel, since it will merely generate a new host of unusual problems. There may be a break-in period in which you can observe someone else in action; but since direction is a uniquely personal human activity, one model cannot serve all situations. So observe and take notes but do not then, or later, attempt to change departmental standard operating procedures (SOP's) until you have a well-thought-out strategy. Any precipitate action will, in the target (personnel) of your attention, merely arouse reverberating confusion and consternation and perhaps incite either passive or open rebellion. That is more likely to happen with the more senior members who are only marginally competent, especially if the changes proposed are at variance with their abilities.[20]

You may find certain personnel using all their resources to frustrate your direction for change, even to going over your head and appealing to other physicians, the administration, or the union. So you must build the need for improvement as the foundation for change and incorporate all affected members in the development of the solution.

Proceeding full steam ahead without the prior cooperation of departmental personnel will merely lead to showdowns in which there are no winners. Announcing an impending improvement in department services that then fails to materialize (unless you can deliver the product single-handedly) will increase neither your status nor your influence in the hospital. So as leader you must learn to recognize the first signs of an impending stalemate so that you can divert your energies to activity more conducive to bettering the department's performance and enhancing its prestige. Otherwise, you may end up wading through a continuous layer of resistance that is useful only to give you pause after you have moved to some other institution and are tempted to repeat the same assault on protocol. Thus you must learn to discriminate between dead-end situations that can only result in fiasco, situations in which, to be an effective leader of men, you must really do your homework, and those rare instances in which everyone was already going your way.

After a few such experiences the less adaptable director will concentrate on areas of service that he can personally accomplish unaided. Now the repertoire of that specialty may contain specific medical techniques that need to be performed repeatedly by the director. However, if as the leader you overly often perform a series of medical technical activities that others present could also perform, you will soon create the stereotype that you are a technician rather than a leader.[21] While it is important, as part of the basis for your leadership, to provide technical expertise, it is only a part of that basis, as we discussed previously. If indeed you are being paid to direct as well as for the use of your name (license) and your expertise (techniques), then such a narrowing of your focus will certainly be noted and perhaps acted upon in a manner adverse to your interests.

HOW TO BUILD A TEAM

One role that no effective leader should delegate is that of scrutinizing and approving prospective members of the department. In some hospitals the supervisors have assumed this role (operational team leader by default?), so that it may no longer be your prerogative or problem. Nevertheless, legally and functionally it is a potential pitfall, since you are ultimately responsible for the product of employee performance. If you also consider that each time you hire an individual you are committing the hospital to a potential investment, if he or she stays ten years or more, of between $80,000 and $150,000, a searching examination of the candidate is obviously mandatory. No director in his right mind would ever order a piece of capital equipment in that price range with the cursory review usually given to most "new hires."

The nature of the selection process is determined by the definition of the opening. If the opening is for a team member, then the applicant should fit team criteria. Too often choices based upon misconceptions of the position lead to an ever-widening array of problems. The basic element of the hospital organization is the team. A team is a group of people with a common purpose who, in spite of their operationally important individual differences, can be so coordinated that their synergistic effort culminates in a result that supersedes the sum of individual actions.[22]

> Group members learn new ways of relating to one another in the organizational context which are likely to increase group effectiveness. . . . Team building is important because the group is helped to identify and change various group norms and patterns of interpersonal relationships.[23]

Thus to mold this amalgam of unique individuals into a coherent whole, you must have a clear conception of what elements to seek. Sampson succinctly itemized the essential elements in assembling an ideal work group. Adapted for the hospital situation they are as follows:[24]

1. Acceptance of the department's purpose, both overt and covert, by the medical director. No such problem exists in the traditional departments. However, I have witnessed numerous instances of cross-purposes in the therapeutically oriented departments that have reduced group effectiveness dramatically.

2. A corollary acceptance of the medical director by his department staff. The problem here has two components: (a) Does the director have the special training that clearly makes him eligible for the post? (b) What is his credibility as a responsible leader? Deficiencies in either area may presage future problems, but most staffs will initially give him the benefit of the doubt unless, of course, the former leader is still on the scene.

3. Sufficient time together to develop a coherent group entity after someone has set about building a team in an effective manner.

4. Channels of communication adequate for the group's purpose. Delivery of information hours or days later is as deleterious as the withholding of information. Most events and their appropriate response have a built-in time priority.

5. Team assets. Obviously, to be effective, the members must be competent. Thus there cannot be too great a disparity between the highest and lowest levels; if there is, the two cannot properly support each other in the group's task.

6. Compatibility is essential to personnel working in a crisis environment. The most technically superior member of the group, if not accepting of the group, will be nearly ineffectual in teamwork situations. Thus there must be enough give and take that group activity is agreeable and rewarding.

7. A commitment to a goal acceptable to all in that hospital. If the greater purpose is each individual's welfare, that will quickly weaken unity and effectiveness. In fact, it is possible to develop goals contrary to the institution's goals. Many of these are secondary and unspoken and will need to be publicly examined to be resolved.

8. Trust, based upon credibility and consistency, that the director and team must generate each and every day. Once serious misgivings emerge about group purpose or effectiveness, the vicious cycle of the self-fulfilling prophecy is triggered. Only radical action will avert disaster.

9. Mutual support—each member to the degree of his or her commitment to the group will be appropriately supportive of group functions and goals regardless of the reason for any current deficiency.

10. Candor in interpersonal relations—there are likely to be many times when emotionally charged material is generated in a crisis situation. The situation must be handled in a fashion supportive of the group and should result in group influence upon individual behavior as needed. Members must be free to provide supportive and constructive activity to regain group norms.

11. Development of shared leadership in each task signals a maturation of the group. These "informal leaders"[25] spontaneously assume responsibility as the situation demands without regard to the organizational structure of the department.

If you are a latecomer to the scene, you should analyze the existing team's performance based upon these criteria. In this socially protective era one cannot casually discard the incumbents and restaff the department to his own tastes. The first target of your study should be the current supervisor unless the administration is willing to transfer him laterally in order to free up the position for your man. In such an event you must be even more thorough in your observations and more circumspect in your early manipulations of the group.

THE SUPERVISOR

Again the options are determined by your specialty. In the regulated departments (Radiology and Laboratory/Pathology) there is a well-demarcated road to the supervisor's position: Training programs turn out consistent products from which are drawn those with the drive and determination to either work their way up from the ranks or enlist in various "management for supervisory personnel" training programs. Normally, survivors of this rigorous obstacle course are quite competent; and as long as they are prepared to accept you as the medical director, you should have few problems. However, you must be wary in your initial attempts to establish rapport with the department personnel not to present the appearance of a threat to the supervisor's authority.

In the less regular departments the situation is not quite so clear, since formal training for the post is rudimentary. There are quite a few basic situations, and you should quickly decide which of them is most applicable.

Situation 1. The supervisor is competent, experienced, and willing to accept you on your terms as director. But you must discriminate this from the converse situation: the superficially competent supervisor with a gift for blarney whose flattery is designed to disarm you and keep you from discovering his inadequacies. If you can get around the facade skillfully, perhaps you can help him.

Situation 2. Here the supervisor is marginally competent but is so well ensconced in the management power structure (seniority, political affiliations, and union) that early attempts to replace him will be stalemated. This will be a long pull, so you should study the man to determine the possibly remediable or irremediable aspect: (1) deficiency due to prior inadequate medical direction, which you can correct, (2) technical deficiencies that, with your stimulus and his drive, can be corrected, (3) human relations management problems that you can perhaps supplement, or (4) low rating on all levels without ability to allow improvement. If in the last instance you elect to drive him out, you may just possibly have committed yourself to a five-year program.

Situation 3. There is no supervisor in the department. Medical staff and administration alike look to you to provide the best. Your survey of the department staff fails to turn up anyone with real potential but does excite interest in those with most seniority on the basis of "It's my turn now." In the absence of obviously superior, and affordable, talent, you can appoint an acting supervisor, but you must specify the term of say three months unless a permanent choice can be found sooner. It is essential that you interview in depth and perhaps repeatedly the available candidates to get a feeling for what is available. Consult with any school/ society/association of the discipline for job description and recommendations. Refrain from attempting to hire someone away from another position. First, the same person may perform differently under other circumstances, particularly if his professional status is not the same at the second location. Second, luring someone from his job, however indirectly, may put you into an obligatory position that may be embarrassing if the person does not work out. Let him volunteer!

Situation 4. The Chief appoints you, his assistant, to be medical director of the department but conveys a different message, via body language, to the supervisor. There ensues a charade in which, if the supervisor is polite, he may ask you your opinion *before* saying "But Doctor M says. . . ." There is likely to be a large element of loyalty for the Emeritus Director. Thus beset from above and below, you are in a no-win situation. To achieve an equilibrium, dramatic remedies will be required, such as an extended vacation for the Emeritus Director.

Since the majority of supervisors attained their rank by having both adequate technical and human relations ability and by being on board early in the development of the department, their basic management skills may be quite rudimentary. You need to observe their reaction in a crisis involving a sudden shortage of department personnel. If their response is to drop their managerial roles and become technicians fulfilling excess standard demand, you have a moderate, possibly remediable, problem.

If a supervisor performs only the unusual and urgent services but devotes as much attention to seeking more trained help, you can relax. But if he cannot accommodate to crisis and stays frozen in his usual pattern, you had best begin plotting a strategy of replacement. Often the latter type survives by the efforts of his subordinates, who rise to the occasion. But as the informal leaders grow more experienced and effective, they also become threatening and are encouraged to leave by having their freedom of action severely restricted. The index of the supervisor's insecurity is the emotion he displays on announcing a departure—even at a most inopportune time for the department.

THE MANAGEMENT OF CONFLICT

The prime cause of conflict often lies in past events. If a dynamic supervisor has had to make do with minimal or no medical supervision until your appointment and you intend to take your responsibilities seriously, then a clash is certain. He will look to you only when expanding those activities that require a medical license, and he will keep the rest under his total control. He has built up the administrative and medical staff liaison and backup from before. He will certainly have a good working knowledge of the politics. And, most importantly, not realizing the limitations of his single, nonmedical background approach, he will resist promptly and effectively when you attempt to introduce a different and better way of doing things. So if you respond automatically to his answering push with an increased shove, the struggle will be on. You must proceed by first acquainting him with the broader background of the events you wish to see brought about. Otherwise, he will merely attempt to manipulate you with all of the various mechanisms that he has perfected in his years of practice on the medical staff.

If you choose to act precipitately, before you have reconnoitered the situation, you may find that you, not he, are under attack. First, he has had a long history of an effective working relation with the hospital but you are a new and unknown factor. Second, his input to and contact with administration will exceed yours by a factor of ten. Third, until you have had the time to demonstrate your worth to the medical staff, he is likely to continue to have equal influence. Fourth, he can reduce the input you need to be effective during the initial period when you have no alternative sources. A clever way of doing that subtly is to remove the time pressure on delivery of information so that you always seem to hear about acute needs too late to respond with maximal effectiveness.

As the director struggles in this confusion but also finds that, when he acts as a physician, everything proceeds smoothly, his normal response will be to concentrate on medical activities. On the other hand, if when he tries to involve himself in department affairs he is frustrated but can gather no evidence of deliberate misconduct, he is being emotionally conditioned by aversion therapy. Thus he will gradually withdraw from the situations in which he is ill at ease in preference to those in which he can feed his self-esteem. Thus the director, by his automatic response to such pressures, may find his major focus shifted to patient contact activities. Since no one is challenging his legal and financial claims on the directorship, he may tacitly accept the new assignment and become a staunch supporter of his manipulative supervisor.

Flippo devotes an entire chapter to this one problem for those who wish more detail. He concludes with a pragmatic summation that is the most realistic approach for the director with this problem.[26]

> The classical management approach is to rely on the first method, where either party must win or lose. The modern behavioral approach suggests that, where mutual trust and genuine human relationships have been established, the last approach can be used. Under the win/win approach to conflict resolution, it is assumed that the conflict is caused by relationships among people and not within the person; rarely is one party completely right and the other completely wrong; and finally, granting concessions is not a sign of weakness.

ONGOING SUPERVISION

In spite of the preceding recital of difficulties, the great majority of departmental supervisors and personnel are adequate to the task at hand. To maintain course, particularly when conditions are changing, the director must exert regular and routine control that should, in addition, fulfill legal obligations. Since the potentially most highly variable element in the department is the performance of the personnel, it should be given the highest priority.

Many activities are semi-independent; that is, no other member of the department is available when that service is performed. But there will be observers—patients, other hospital personnel, and physicians—so a large part of ongoing control consists in maintaining the broadest possible net for any information pertaining to your personnel in discharge of their duty. You must develop some method of determining level of competence on a regular, repetitive basis. Personal observations, by you and the supervisor, of activities is only one aspect. Objective criteria of adequacy *and* relevancy of service should also be developed, since you will ultimately need them to satisfy fiscal intermediaries who demand proof that they got what they paid for. For those technical areas that lack any external control, Public Law 92-603 has established a mechanism out of which will arise nationwide validating, certifying, and regulating activities.

You must, therefore, evolve a written policy that outlines the various levels of supervision as a group, as individuals, and as task-related. Annual informal reviews of each member's performance when merit increases are being considered barely satisfy some of the requirements. A checklist type of task analysis based upon the job description would be more appropriate. One resource in this supervision that is commonly overlooked is that of the employees themselves. Let the people doing the jobs participate in developing criteria of adequate performance for each task. Here your skillful guidance and broader viewpoint will be essential.

IN-SERVICE TRAINING

Administrators expect appropriate efforts to keep their hospital services current and competitive. That implies some form of continuing education. The personnel policy of the hospital also may require such efforts if the practice is to hire the least expensive talent and upgrade it on the job. That can be a short-sighted approach insuring increased turnover because skills and experience accumulate faster than commensurate fiscal returns. So as the initially marginal employee improves to adequate levels, he or she may then seek a higher-salaried position elsewhere. As a result the wide recurrent variation in the quality of departmental services casts a shadow on the reputation of the department.

Although in-service educational efforts are a vital community service and provide much job benefit, the hospital's primary function is health care for patients, not a training station for staff on their way to better opportunities. Through misdirected emphasis on economy at top policy levels, and a corollary emphasis on quality control at the middle level, too much effort may be expended on education at the expense of patient care. According to formal school regulations, hospital affiliates cannot reduce their normal staffing to take advantage of the presence of students. However, when the "student" is merely a raw recruit or part of a class from a commercial school, such regulations are ignored. The director and, more importantly, the patients are left with a pool of talent sadly inadequate to the day-to-day needs.

Again the wide range of educational resources and requirements makes useful specification difficult. Certainly in areas with adequate regulations and entrance requirements the professional societies and the manufacturers will provide this function adequately. But in areas in which numbers are few and formal requirements scanty, the major burden will fall on the director. In an effort to reduce the load by subcontracting, the director may fall into the trap of "the multiplicative effects of repeated transcription error."

The scenario, based upon the venerable principle of "see one, do one, teach one," is as follows: The new director teaches Joe the routine of department tasks and services but fails to insure Joe's understanding of the basic principles upon which those activities are based. As the director's and Joe's load increases, Sam is hired and Joe is delegated to show him the ropes. Subsequently Sam teaches Paul, who teaches Bill, who teaches George, who teaches Allan. One day someone expert in the field watches Allan perform his duties in a way that leads to results far different from those originally intended. If it is the original director, he will be horrified and start a witch hunt for the one who perpetrated this bastardy. If it is a new associate of the director, the affair will merely confirm his suspicions that the Chief is inadequate. If it is a medical staff member, he will now be certain that the department exists only to make money, not provide service. So the director, to protect his own interests, as well as those of the department, must set up a system that will not allow deviation from established norms.

VALUE OF HUMAN RESOURCES

Directors have an amazing dichotomy in their approach to the two most expensive items in their departments: personnel and major capital equipment. Selecting a $25,000 piece of equipment from among two or three brands will require hours of consideration, days of indecision, phone calls to colleagues who have used it or them, careful reading of the literature, and quite possibly clinical trials. An employee who stays three years will cost that much, if not more with benefits, yet directors are proud that they spend a cursory fifteen minutes with each applicant. We obviously have been conditioned to consider equipment more important and prestigious than trained human talent. In comparison, how often do you hear someone bragging about his new machine compared to a new talent?

Having assigned a lower order of priority to personnel, we then magnify any problems by the way in which we conduct our interviews. Most interviews follow no coherent pattern and vary from applicant to applicant. Some institutions pride themselves on the fact that they "give an exam," yet most surveys of quality control disclose that errors were due primarily to the lack of application of known facts rather than to an absence of critical information. The erring person, fully aware of the necessary information, persists in ill-advised activity. Thus, testing the applicant for depth of knowledge is no guarantee that he will use his knowledge to good purpose.

Yet the predominant approach to hiring personnel is to try to acquire the least expensive talent on the ground that this approach is more effective in cost control. But if optimum service and fiscal

Table 1. Relative value of personnel of XYZ service at hospital ABC.

	Entry Level Skill		
	I	II	III
Basic entry salary*	$745/mo.	$890/mo.	$940/mo.
Specific skills of applicant	A,B,C,D, E,F,G,H,I	A,B,C,D, E,F,G,H, I,J,K,L, M,N,O,P,Q	A,B,C,D, E,F,G,H, I,J,K,L, M,N,O,P, Q,R,S,T, U,V,W,X, Y,Z
Value of services person can perform under normal load	$1,005/wk.	$2,165/wk.	$2,596/wk.
Value of routine work ordered that person cannot perform	$1,591/wk.	$ 431/wk.	$ 0/wk.
Personnel cost of first month orientation and in-service to assure quality	$ 562	$ 450	$ 217

*Based upon minimal acceptable experience.

solvency are indeed the hospital's credo, it will never be served by hiring a predominance of the lowest-level talent. Table 1 shows a survey that was conducted at one hospital and was intended to impress the fiscal authority with the illogic of seeking the lowest common denominator. From a pragmatic point of view, selecting personnel with experience is the wisest course for one major reason: They have probably committed their major mistakes elsewhere. That is exactly what schools are for; they provide an artificial environment in which errors and blunders can be committed without real cost. Additionally, one would hope that there is a record of each individual's learning curve to help you in your evaluation of his or her past and potential track record.

It is essential that you have the specific job description for each applicant you interview. It not only lists the tasks and skills that the position calls for but should also set forth clearly and specifically what kind of person is needed to do the job. All that should be spelled out in as much detail as possible: educational requirements, skill requirements, human relations ability, test scores, experience, and physical characteristics. Since the individual is to work in a "crisis environment" dealing with a variety of people, it is especially important to determine if he or she is capable of listening, comprehending, communicating, reading, calculating, and thinking logically. Not all high school diplomas are equal even if the law says they are. Too often we are misled by dress, appearance, and manner and fail to check the basic operational aspects of a potential employee.

SALARIES

Although theoretically salaries are the sole concern of the supervisor and hospital administration, the practical fact is that the director also must be aware of the situation. Who is getting what and why? Government regulations forbid a differential between two individuals doing the same job except on the basis of (1) seniority and (2) added training and responsibility. Otherwise, one must suspect favoritism. That is particularly important if different employees progress up the scale at a rate different from that of their overall performance. Also, in competing for scarce talent, one must know where he stands in relation to other hospitals in order to work out fringe benefits that may make the crucial difference.

Ideally, the hospital must pay the prevailing community level of wages and salaries. Factors such as productivity, union pressure, and wages paid by competitors for similar services are major considerations in wage and salary deliberations. It is desirable to conduct wage surveys through the Personnel Department so that each organization can acquire factual information about wages currently paid in its labor market. However, a wide discrepancy often exists between what an organization does and what it says it does in wage policy. Equitable wage and salary distribution within the organization is established through the Personnel Department by job evaluation: a process of studying job descriptions and job specifications to determine levels of responsibility and difficulty of job performance that can be translated into pay scales. Job evaluation provides consistent, equitable wage and salary distribution within the organization at the paperwork level.

DEPLOYMENT TO MEET DEMAND

Every successful director will ultimately arrive at a time when he must demand more of his staff than they can deliver. Essentially that is a problem of too few people to meet the demand. The crisis may arise because department coverage is extended to more than one shift, success of educational drive increases the number of requests for service, or key people leave or fall ill and lag time to replacement is too long. The dilemma will be this: do you use partly trained, marginally competent people (second string) or do you push your top line to work longer hours? The latter course may merely lead to further shortage in succeeding days. At this point you can never be certain that you have adequate coverage, and the medical staff will not be reluctant to complain. The saving grace, politically, is that most of the medical and nursing staff cannot tell the difference between marginally good and marginally bad services. However, you and, especially, your staff will know the difference, and it will not enhance morale and may actually promote further losses.

Your solution is to try to recruit extra help from other institutions, but you are likely to find that the others are doing the same thing. Contrary to popular notions, most health workers expect reasonable hours of work and regular time off for their personal affairs. If you yourself cannot set an example during this crisis, you may find it increasingly difficult to squeeze the extra hours and effort out of your staff. At this point you may be tempted to accede to many irregular solutions ranging from significant erosion of quality of service to use of inadequate personnel. You may even lose more experienced personnel whose professionalism is affronted—and who know of increased job opportunity elsewhere. Apart from having enough staff and reserves in the first place, one approach is to combine resources of several institutions in in-service training to upgrade marginal talent. Also, any minor surplus of part-time people can be more efficiently used to meet vagaries of demand. But you should be certain that wage and hours regulations are properly observed. An employee on detached duty is still entitled to extra credit for hours in excess of 80 in a pay period. If the demand is seasonal, you have a breathing space in which to make more appropriate plans for next time. In that interim you must intensify recruiting, selection, training, and pruning.

SEPARATION

To work effectively as a team, your staff members must be compatible. One manifestation of compatibility is acceptance of group goals. Those who do not accept group goals—aptly labeled peripheral employees by M. J. Gannon[27]—are unable to accommodate to any unusual demand such as working overtime, learning new skills, changing shifts, or working extra time. Legally you are obligated to give each employee a fair chance to measure up before separation should be considered. More often than not, separation occurs voluntarily among those you would prefer to keep and bypasses those you would love to lose. That happens because of various intangibles in the interaction process previously mentioned. Whatever the reason, if employees become unhappy enough—sufficiently to lose their sense of identity with the team—to look elsewhere, you can anticipate eventual departure. That is particularly apt to happen if the director or supervisor indulges in his or her own strong ego feelings in the form of reprimand during times of stress. The costs of departures are considerable and are suggested by the following factors:

—When in the eyes of the department staff employees, X is dismissed without just cause, employee morale and efficiency may drop.

—Hospital payment toward unemployment compensation is based upon an experience rating procedure.

—High turnover gives a department a bad image and impairs recruitment.

—Excessive discharges imply that the leader is incapable of properly selecting, training, and motivating employees.

—There is a real cost to recruiting and selecting a replacement.

—There is a dollar cost to training a replacement.

—There is the loss of revenues for services ordered but never performed.

—The replacement is overpaid during break-in period when he or she cannot perform at full efficiency.

—Overtime work will be put in by others during the hiatus.

—There is a potential cost of failure to maintain or utilize equipment during the training period.

To discharge an employee, you must give him due process as outlined in the labor code—repeated warning in writing, counseling, review, attempt at rehabilitation, then firing. There are a host of other methods of causing an employee to split; most supervisors are aware of their existence and their questionable legality. As long as other job openings exist, problems leading to formal complaint will be rare. Personnel journals contain numerous studies of all those aspects and are a good source of specific information.

MOTIVATION

Dr. Oh neatly describes motivation:[28]

There are numerous motivation theories, but they can be roughly divided into two approaches to motivating workers. One school of thought is based on the assumption that man can be motivated through external factors such as money, security, etc.—i.e., tangible factors. Another school of thought supposes that man can be successfully motivated through intangible, internal factors such as a challenging job, personal growth, satisfaction through recognition, etc. However, if any single conclusion can be drawn from a review of motivation theories, it is that there is no single management strategy that will work for all men at all times under all conditions. The worker himself is extremely complex and highly variable in the pattern of his motivations. In addition to intra- and interpersonal variations in motivational patterns, a manager, in devising his management strategies, must also deal with the variety in the kinds of tasks they perform. Any one approach could be wrong for some workers under some conditions.

In order to be successful, a manager must first be an inquisitive and sensitive diagnostician of the differences in ability and motivation among the people who work for him. And he must value rather than deplore these differences. Finally, he must have the flexibility and wide repertoire of management skills to adapt himself to the differences and to function in a variety of interpersonal and psychological relationships and authority patterns.

Whatever approach that you as a director use in assembling and forging your team, a key principle is that your work is never done. When a concrete structure is under way, a stage of completion is reached; the builder can step aside and the structure persists. In contrast, an organizational structure requires the same level of effort and attention downstream as it did in the initial phases. Thus once you stop leading, you will find that the balance of forces in the organization changes. There are no successful part-time leaders—leading is a full-time job.

4

THE
OPERATIONAL
FUNCTION

SOLVENCY AND SURVIVAL

No one, not even the administrator, can long remain on the payroll of a bankrupt organization—unless, of course, it is tax-supported. Consequently, the administrator will expect each potentially profitable department to pay its way. He certainly will look with disfavor on tactics that may erode a department's positive fiscal position. Thus the director must be cognizant of all factors that influence the balance sheet, including incurred costs, efficiency, and level of utilization.

About 60 percent of the monies expended in providing hospital care goes to personnel. Capital costs are equally important, since a bad choice may, in effect, not only close off the possibility of cost recovery but also result in the loss of potentially more desirable options. Also, responding to pressures by the administrator and department supervisor, and the director's own contractual obligation, will subtly motivate actions that will enhance increasing utilization. An optimum way to cope with this complex input is to adopt a systems approach in operational management. That means you must develop a viewpoint that allows you to consider and

handle all the varied interrelated and interdependent elements of
your complex situation.[29]

The director's appropriate response to increasing demand is to
confirm the department's ability to cope with the growing need. Is
the department adequately staffed and equipped and able to perform in concert with other hospital services? For maximal effectiveness its facilities and resources must be at the same level of
development as the rest of the hospital's services. Too great a disparity in either direction will merely generate accessory problems.
Does the department meet optimum community standards? Again,
if the disparity is negative and goes uncorrected, it will result in a
shift of patients to other hospitals. A significant fiscal consequence
will then arise from submaximal operations. The director, therefore, will find himself acting as broker between the desires of the
administrator and the department, the needs of the medical staff,
and the implicit demands of the patients served.

The problem may be heightened by the nature of the director's
own contractual agreement with the hospital. If the director should
promote utilization beyond the effectiveness of delivery or condone
a downward revision in quality of product, he may be taken to
task. State medical societies have been scrutinizing the details of
contractual agreements between physician and hospital, and now
the third-party payers are evincing growing interest. Logically, the
ultimate answer is for the director to insure the best attainable
quality of product *and* promote a competently trained medical staff
who will use the services appropriately and correctly. That is a
rather tall order. When looking at the operational aspects of department function, one must realize that he will be judged for results, not good intentions, and consequently will be responsible for
unanticipated problems even though unwillingly shared.

THE LANGUAGE OF MANAGEMENT

The key to success in the management process is to
make decisions based upon pertinent, adequate, and objective
feedback. To perceive things the way they are rather than the way
you want them to be is critical to effective decision making. Thus

you will find that all precise disciplines rely heavily upon the written word. In medicine, although we record a tremendous amount of data on patients, a major part of the communication volume upon which decisions are based is purely verbal and hence subjective. That approach is not acceptable in the management process. In the words of Pfifner and Sherwood,[30]

> Organizations are bound by impersonal rules, and this binding contributes to stability and predictability of behavior among members. Also, members of organizations have assigned tasks based on their areas of competence, which gives the advantage of specialization. This also contributes to predictability of behavior. In addition, all administrative actions are bounded by rules and are recorded permanently, which also contributes to stability and predictability. Thus, the emphasis on forms, records and reporting, and hierarchy, controls all units of the organization. However, this very rationality of organization has often been a source of potential conflict and frustration.

No administrator can personally supervise and comprehend the intent of each facet of his complex hospital organization. Thus he must rely upon delegated subordinates—specialists and supervisors—to reduce the operations of their departments to a common format on paper. To control, the administrator demands data in a form from which he can make "maps of the territory" his organization is traversing.

To paraphrase Luthans,[31] bureaucratic organizations require written records of all actions taken and decisions made and the data sources upon which they are based. That provides standardization and, in cases of recurring problems, the predictability from past actions preserved in written memory. Records and reports, in addition to providing justification for action, serve to extend control to areas one cannot physically supervise. The real plague of paperwork is due to neglect of two essential elements: purpose and timeliness. As long as the record is pertinent to the problem rather than generated to serve some subsidiary goals, it should be prepared. The information contained must be timely, up-to-date, and accurate. Ideally, each report, unless a data sheet, should have an expiry date similar to that on a pharmaceutical.

To the medical director the most frustrating aspect of communicating in the language of management is the necessity of writing everything he wishes to say. That is particularly distressing to specialists whose fact and opinion categories have ill-defined boundaries. Thus to be effective, someone in the department must grind out the requisite data and projections and recommendations on paper to fulfill administration's need for input. Since most directors would be horrified to have that as part of their job descriptions, they readily delegate it to subordinates.

The growing fiscal intermediary and government involvement in health care has further accentuated the demand for paper talk each day. The problem is again one of delegation without supervision. It is necessary that the director be aware that the person writing the reports thereby attains status. His selection and output should be scanned, since this output often will have more concrete operational significance than anything that arises from the director's verbal contact with administration.

All departments are in true competition on paper for administrative assistance in planning, operational and capital fund allocation, and so on. Reports that are delayed or incomplete or contain discoverable errors may lead to change in the way the department operates. The change is most apt to occur when the supervisor is problem- rather than goal-oriented and hence, during a staff shortage crisis, pitches in with department services and abandons essential paperwork. That, although commendable from the idealistic point of view, is not prudent management. Departmental income and staffing depend as much upon completion of the necessary paperwork as upon demand for services. Your recourse, then, is to appoint someone else to see that the reports and data sheets go in on schedule. If you can oversee the written output, you will quickly gain a clearer picture of what is going on—in addition to fulfilling your legal obligations.

Careful attention to paperwork documenting the need for expansion of sevices will also improve your prospects of attaining your own long-range goals. Administrators, as a matter of course, assume that every director is overly ambitious when he proposes expansion. To the degree that you fail to document the need you profess to serve, you confirm that suspicion. That is particularly true if, early in your career, you did wheedle some expensive equipment that turned out to be disappointing in performance and cost recovery. The administrators will see that item in the yearly report of the department and be guided accordingly. The only hospitals that can potentially afford to neglect cost considerations in expansion are those with a significant outside income or support from the public treasury.

THE DIRECTOR'S INPUT INTO OPERATIONS

The critical element in the director's input into operations is not the degree of involvement, but the degree of *success* of the involvement in departmental operations. The personality and management style of the administrator are of paramount importance here. Some administrators will deal directly only with the department supervisor and almost totally bypass the director no matter how much he may wish to be involved. Then the director's only recourse is to work through the supervisor if he wishes to share in control. Other administrators insist that the director be directly involved either because they are Type Y or because they want the M.D. to be aware of the activities that generate the income that supports him.

The director also makes an operational choice. He may restrictively select the role of technical adviser and ignore departmental function except to complain about personnel, equipment, and special facilities. Most supervisors will accommodate that role, since their own freedom of action is correspondingly greater. Others, realizing the advantage of the M.D.'s broader viewpoint, will attempt to manipulate the director into greater involvement—if only in equipment selection and in-service education. The alternative by which all three—administrator, supervisor, and director—work together in full cooperation and to the maximal advantage of the hospital is obviously the ideal. There still are, on the other hand, a few absentee landlord directors who, having once secured an advantageous agreement with the hospital, subcontract the job to a more junior and less expensive assistant and fade from the daily scene. Obviously such a directorship is a business and not a profession.

Under ideal circumstances the medical director is concerned with the broader aspects of the problem. He educates and is educated by the supervisor, and together, as a team, they evolve more realistic long-range proposals for administrative approval. With the input from the director's medical staff connections and the technical expertise of the supervisor, they rework and modify department services to increase efficiency, reliability, and relevancy.

Now if the department provides therapeutic as well as diagnostic services, the probability that the director's efforts on its behalf will be successful is greatly increased. If the director is involved in patient care and by his efforts can reduce mortality, then those efforts will add a new dimension to his effect upon the department's activity. A prime example, because of its very incidence, is cardiac disease. If the hospital has a yearly admission rate of 200 acute myocardial infarctions with past mortality of about 45 and the new director consultant is able to reduce the mortality to 30, then multiple benefits appear. The 15 who might have otherwise perished early now go on to recovery in 14 to 28 days, and the majority are likely to return again as patients in the future. The efforts, therefore, have likely insured an additional minimum of 200 patient days. Since that effect is, to a degree, multiplicative, utilization of the department and ancillary services increases over succeeding years. Additionally, if word of the improved care gets out to the community, more doctors and patients may be attracted to the hospital.

Of course, when such enhanced activities become widespread, they will ultimately raise a philosophical issue. Since physicians are programmed for one task only, that of "prolonging any useful life," the problems will first have to be worked out at a different level. The prime example currently is the impact that monitoring, Coronary Care Units, and widespread use of antiarrythmic agents have had on acute cardiac mortality. Equal improvements in mortality are occurring in Nephrology and Gastroenterology.

Any such improved care under the guidance of a skilled medical

Table 2. *Costs of hospital treatment of myocardial infarction.*

Year	Average Hospital Stay in Days	Daily Dollar Cost of Hospital Care	Total Cost	Average Mortality Rate
1920	56	$ 3.21	$ 180.00	40%
1930	42	$ 5.00	$ 210.00	30%
1970	28	$125.00	$3500.00	18%

Source: J. H. Knowles, "The Hospital," *Scientific American*, Vol. 293 (1973), No. 3, pp. 128-137.

director will eventually adversely affect the cost experience of the fiscal intermediaries, whose planning and expectations are based upon a far different level of care. The effects on costs are shown in Table 2. Since 1920, 1930, and 1970 dollars are not equivalent, the cost disparity is not as great as it would seem, but on the other hand, many more people now survive to the "coronary age," and so absolute numbers are greater. However, the potential impact of an effective medical director in the clinical specialties is growing greater by the year. If the director is a dynamic and astute teacher so that overall care in his specialty is improved on all fronts, then the long-term effects will be even greater. Since such benefits have their effects on all departments, impetus is provided for closer coordination between all clinical department heads. No one stands to lose by the others' successes in this area.

However, in spite of statistics and theory, problems of control still exist. A case in point is the following: Utilization of Department A in Hospital Z was declining slowly in spite of the best efforts of its director. The problem was that he refused to admit that anyone could be dissatisfied with the services as they were. Because of his close relation with the administrator, he could persistently refuse to allow available and competent peer talent to also use the department. The result was that his fellow specialists set up a competing department in another hospital, listened to the gripes of the practicing physicians, and modified the services to suit the ultimate consumer.

Finally, in response to pressures from his supporters, the original director recruited a dynamic young associate. Together they convinced administration that the answer to the previous "no problem" was to acquire automated equipment and expand into other areas. Contrary to expectation, utilization continued to fall, since what the complaining doctors wanted was an improvement in philosophy of service—not new equipment for a subgroup of their patients. Other departments suffered by having their capital requirements slashed to provide the funds to transfuse Department A's operations. Consequently, equipment update and replacement in other departments was delayed, and the hospital's competitive position was further reduced. These complex political and economic problems ultimately led to open acrimony in the power group but no solution. Thus a minor variation in definition of adequate service by the director, who was in a key power position, led to a cascading series of problems without apparent final solution.

MARKET SURVEY

Having determined what the administration, medical staff, and department are all about in terms of structure, interrelation, and operation, the director should repeat the study from a different perspective. He should examine the basic assumptions from which departmental activity originates. Otherwise, he could follow the same track until he runs up against a stone wall of demand altered by technological and social change. Who are the large-volume users of the department and what is their medical background? What do they see as present and as future needs? Are they aware of the major technological trends on the horizon? What will be the impact of those changes on them? Or do they all plan to retire before such changes occur? If so, is anyone preparing to seek replacement?

It might be useful to study the age and specialty distribution of the entire active medical staff and even plot such trends as the number of new applicants accepted and the number resigning each year. The same patient problem is often perceived in a different light by physicians at different stages of their careers. All those factors will have an effect upon the present and future pattern of utilization.

What of the wider community from which hospital patients are drawn? What is the age distribution, and what are the other relevant demographic factors? The quickest way to obtain these data is to spend some time with the business editor of the local newspaper and the managers of the larger commercial banks. They have data for every year and may be able to display significant trends that will even influence your own future plans. Discuss the findings with the hospital's business manager; for he may be able to draw more practical conclusions from the demographic data, the economic prospects of the area, and the pattern of utilization of the hospital. Even the distribution of the various health insurance plans among patients will point out areas of low or high opportunity. Unless you deliver a very standard product, all of the above information should result in a more refined approach to services, particularly if you can disseminate the findings and implications to your peers.

PAPERWORK

Now that we have directly related medical care to economics, we should examine channels of communication. The various fiscal intermediaries require documentation of services ordered and delivered, and in some cases the quality of service, before paying the charges generated. Thus the data will have to go out on a daily basis to keep administration and business office current. But that is only a small segment of the ongoing departmental record-keeping activity. Although the director need not read every piece of paper, he should be aware of the existence of all the record categories maintained so that, in case of need, he knows the material is available.

The running record of department business, in response to public regulations and administrative needs, must encompass every official activity. The portions of concern to the director are the procedure manuals, which detail each activity and how and when it should be done, the in-service records, and the files on individual employees. A manual not only is required for accreditation but is also a formal channel of input into departmental procedure. If you wish any task changed, that change, to be effective, must appear in the manual. To disseminate the change, there must be an "in-service session" on the topic so the records will reflect compliance. Finally, each employee's file lists his job description, his competency, and the areas in which improvement is needed. You can determine who should be doing what, and whether he is properly prepared. All this is documentation of how well the policies you establish are being implemented.

There are other records with which the medical director is professionally involved. They are the diagnostic activities with his interpretations and comments, and they represent a major reason for the existence of the position. Even here one might reexamine the traditional format to see if there is not a better way to present or deliver the information. With the increased volume of data deluging the physician daily, an improved method of display to the doctor requesting the help may give the advantage you seek.

BUDGETS

At least once a year the director is involved in a major planning project—the budget. There is always a due date, so if you do not receive the request well in advance, you are warned that the supervisor is jamming your channels of communication. The part you play will depend upon how much time you dedicate to the project, and that relates directly to your influence. The type of budget requested will be determined by the philosophy and style of the administrator. Some administrators wish exact numbers in all categories and excessive justification of any capital requests for the next fiscal year. Others require a shade less precision but more input of long-term trends and ask for alternative courses.

To the administrator the budget is the yardstick against which he measures adequacy of planning and performance. In essence, each department extrapolates what it expects to do in the next year from the preceding year's performance. The degree of congruence between a preceding year's budget and actual departmental performance may be an index of planning skill or merely evidence of the small rate of change in utilization. Since no one can accurately prognosticate future events, budgets will always tend to be inaccurate to the degree next year is different from the last.

The rationale of budgets is based upon the validity of prediction from statistical trends. That is most apt to be useful in the areas in which change is slow and regular and can readily be plotted. There you can take the department's preceding year's figures, add x percent, and be smugly certain you will be on target. However, areas undergoing rapid evolution, particularly with significant changes in direction, are less amenable to such easy prediction. There you may be trapped by the intrinsic restrictive nature of the budget process.

Budgets are divided into several categories, and for a complex operation you will have to use them all:[32]

1. Fixed budgets for specific time periods, which do not allow for cost changes. Included are previous amortization, replacement of obsolescent equipment, current space allocation, and basic maintenance and service costs.

2. Flexible budgets, which relate to areas in which major variations are the rule. In the hospital the flexible budget is particularly applicable to personnel costs and supplies and disposables. Here the director and supervisor do have opportunity to analyze the variables and introduce contingency factors. If y increases by 25 percent, then x should be adjusted by $+50$ percent, and so on.

3. Capital budget, which is a major investment designed to maintain, upgrade, or improve service. Here the variability is in the chance for approval. Characteristically, administration requests some sort of priority indexing; it may, for example, want not only the order of priority but also the year in which the item will be required. Since each new major item may require such support as personnel, space, and supplies, this will reflect back to the variable budget.

Hospital budgeting is complicated by the fact that more items tend to be disapproved or postponed than approved. Administrators, because of the records they keep, know that "*urgently* required" equipment often has no significant effect on the department's running record. So, pragmatically, they watch for long-term consistency in new requests. If Department X asks for capital item A in year 1, B in year 2, and C in year 3, then delaying requests by a year or more saves money. Department X is still operating without A, B, or C. If, on the other hand, the director asks for item D in years 1, 2, and 3, the administrator gets the message that the department really does need D, and he may approve it. Medical directors are automatically assumed to be guilty of padding.

The medical director demonstrates his real value when he discerns a forthcoming change that would have escaped the notice of the supervisor, and thereby prevents investment in expensive, but soon to be obsolescent, equipment. Ideally, one should have an alternate contingency plan for each major probability, but generally that is merely an exercise in penmanship. There need be only a broad outline of what may occur and what the appropriate response would be. Unanticipated events and changes are best met without preconceptions as to what they should mean.

Since you will be developing the budget with him, your supervisor will inform you of its format and necessary content. However, you should not pass up an opportunity to discuss the budget with the major users of the service and perhaps more generally with the other directors. In this age of technological acceleration, traditional boundaries are being obliterated, so that there will be more overlapping of services. Thus you need to know who is planning what, and you need to know it well in advance of submitting your final budget version.

That brings us back to the games that administrators play. Ideally there should be a prefinal session in which tentative plans are aired so that relevant feedback results and adjustments are made. At the very least the final budget, board-approved, should be announced to all the medical directors and supervisors so that activity for the next year can be coordinated. If neither session nor announcement occurs and if, in addition, you cannot clearly find out what portion of your budget was approved, you are dealing with a tyrant and not an administrator. Divide to conquer is a technique meant to apply to the enemy. If you find it being used on you, there is only one logical conclusion.

The cat-and-mouse game is often cloaked by a demand for more documentation and feasibility studies, intended to keep you from realizing the truth, lest you react too strongly. Top-level management implies control; but if it is properly exercised, appropriate responsibility is delegated. Certainly if the administrator, without input in open forum from those intimately concerned, is making decisions as to which department he will allow to expand and which not, he is acting in a way that can only be interpreted as punitive and is revealing his own serious management problems.

Unfortunately, administrators also respond to appropriate levels of pressure. If as a consequence objectivity is lost, the decisions are based on friendship, animosity, me-too-ism, and so on. The result is that credibility and full support by medical directors also are lost. In turn, that will result in the director diverting interest and activity to other areas. The administrator will be left with a clear field but without the intangible resources—interest in quality, discernment of trends, opening of new avenues, interest in cost saving—he also needs.

As we have seen, the budget is an excellent tool for both planning and control. It does, however, have some shortcomings. As early as 1953, Chris Argyris identified some human problems that arise from budgets in industrial concerns and perhaps hospitals also. Some of his findings were that budgets tend to unite the lower-echelon people against the hierarchy and create undue tension. Often the tension leads to inefficiency, aggression, and perhaps a complete breakdown in planning on the part of the supervisor. In addition, the use of the budget by top management to needle lower-level personnel tends to make each supervisor see only the problems of his own department rather than the needs and problems of the organization as a whole. [33,34]

GETTING MONEY

Many directors, particularly if their department operations are unusually profitable, act as though surpluses should be devoted exclusively to their departments. They develop budgets based upon the calculated surpluses without realizing that theirs is a beautiful pipe dream. In fact, yelling at the administrator about a badly needed piece of equipment is likely to be more effective than the demand "Why can't we spend what we earn?" The surplus from profitable departments is used to pay the costs of necessary activities that operate at a loss.

However, the absolute degree of profitability does have some effect on the administrative reaction to requests for funds, provided the administrator is not using budget allocation to express approval or disapproval of the department or its director. A director can discuss the potential income that will be lost if the equipment is not obtained, but he can have more impact by pointing out the potential loss of income if patients are sent elsewhere for the service. Since each patient day represents several hundred dollars of income to the hospital, losing a patient to a competing hospital is a real threat. Prolonging patient stay by a day waiting for test results is in another category.

If the situation is truly desperate, the only alternative is to use medical staff action to pry the money loose. You may attempt to do it openly, but unless you are politically astute and possess facts that cannot be interpreted in any other way, you may well lose for any number of reasons not apparent to you. An open confrontation wherein you whip up medical staff support is not conducive to reasoned bargaining. Thus the very manner in which you introduce the business may seal its fate. The other route is to solicit, usually on basis of friendship, some influential doctor to present your case. In doing that, however, you imply that you will henceforth abide by those secret rules, and that is a step you may not wish to take.

The last real alternative is either to go back and develop data and documentation you can present as a valid emergency budget request or to ascertain the leasing cost and present that as an alternate solution, the cost to be paid out of income generated by the equipment.

THE DIVIDE-AND-CONQUER TACTIC

In most hospitals where the administrator – medical staff conflict is below the surface, administrators still react in a manner worthy of some comment. To prevent the theoretical possibility of the medical staff ganging up on them, they go to devious and persistent lengths to promote factionalism. Since the prime threats to their total control are doctors with managerial ability and experience, obviously directors have a high priority as targets.

It is relatively easy to keep departments in competition for space, equipment, and personnel. All that is necessary is to give the major budget allocation to the department whose director has the best record of support of administrative positions. The lesson is not lost on the others, and the directors whose long-range plans are not in step with the administration's find themselves negatively conditioned as they get behind in the capital race. Since budget allocations are made privately, no one knows what the other is asking, only what he is getting. Thus if you try to press for more funds, you have no way to know the reasonableness of the defense "there isn't enough for that this year." Even if it were possible to get all the directors around a table and agree to review all major capital items, the administrator could still play the game on the side. Each time a new piece of major equipment that was never on the agenda appeared, impetus for cooperative action would slacken appreciably.

RELEVANT SERVICES

Since current medical care is a team affair, its various components need to be supportive and harmonious. Yet the spirit of competition or the excessive zeal of one or two men can disrupt the essential balance of departmental services. In the first instance, several hospitals are in competition, and so when one of them suddenly acquires a piece of equipment, the others, under the me-too principle, are compelled to follow suit. Thus capital expenditures are being "decided" by effective salesmanship. This can easily become a vicious cycle that totally wrecks any plan for rational growth. This parochialism is a dynamic force. When augmented by some excess of other emotions, it sweeps all logical argument aside.

In the second situation, a hospital administrator yields to the blandishments of a dynamic subspecialist who claims that, given a free hand, he will make the hospital the center for LMN disease in the community. The plan is to replicate a university-level laboratory in the community hospital. Rather than analyze the local situation and determine what "tests" would be most useful to the specific medical staff, the new director orders the complex and impressive equipment that he had been using at the training institution.

The fact is that medical care at a university center for any common condition is significantly more expensive than at the community hospital level, yet the patient results are equivalent.[35] The reason is that physicians in training order more tests—which may have little influence upon therapy or end results. On the other hand, a university-level lab in a community hospital almost always is underutilized; for the practicing clinician wants short intelligible answers that tell him what to do next.

QUALITY CONTROL

Quality control as a label and popular slogan is rather new, but it has actually been in existence, under different names, in traditional hospital departments for many decades. Each time a radiologist and his medical staff colleagues look at a radiograph, the quality feedback is direct and immediate. A bad film is a bad film, and a series of such films will provoke some positive action. Similarly, in pathology, the custom of multiple readers (sending problem slides around to other colleagues and to the AFIP) again is direct quality control. In anesthesia, as long as the surgeon has input into his choice of "gas passer," the man with poorer results is effectively docked by having fewer cases.

The quality control problem becomes acute when department repertoire and volume increase to the point that the personal scrutiny by the medical director is obviously inadequate. In the newer disciplines in which the director must personally scrutinize, interpret, and sign each item of service (for example, ECG, EEG, and nuclear scans), quality control is not an issue as long as the director is ethical *and* competently trained. The problem arises when the volume of each item of service is so great that effective individual inspection is obviously impractical; this is the area that demands objective measurements of performance of services by tens of thousands of technicians across the United States. Government is moving into this vacuum with its own surveillance and quality control techniques. Although government people seem to have the problems of the diagnostic branch under fair control, that is not true of the therapeutic services aspects of these departments. That area is under beginning study and application of multiple tentative plans of control.

A most direct approach to quality control would be the application of a single encompassing criterion: Would the director utilize his department's services and the appropriate services of the hospital in the event of his own or a close family member's illness? The onus would be on those who answer no; the problem would be to separate the yesses based on assurance and knowledge from those based on ignorance. Unfortunately, this approach cannot be quantitated, but it would be a most interesting study if some group were able to collect data. The simplest way would be to keep a record of where the medical director and his family are hospitalized, particularly for illnesses involving his specialty.

Multiple levels of society are concerned with quality of health care, but that attention is blunted by the greater concern with health care costs. The confusion at this interface presents a golden opportunity for those who provide high volume and whose argument runs, "At such a low unit cost, why bother with extensive quality control?" Yet it is just such high-volume low-quality operations that reward the director in the greatest manner. When one considers the cumulative cost of the mass of these cheap items, the probability of cost overrun becomes apparent.

Third-party payers are now beginning to compare the total costs of care of a specific disease process in all the institutions in a wide area. One such comparison revealed tremendous variation among some institutions. Although undoubtedly difficult to compare, the data are readily amenable to statistical techniques. And who will make sure that the cases are comparable? The PSRO, that's who! Once the various areawide Professional Standards Review Organization (Public Law 92-603) is in full swing, it will be possible to compare the costs of getting the same results at different institutions.

When a director cannot inspect each unit of his department's product, the current method is to use the systems analysis technique. What are the stages of production and delivery that are amenable to quality control methods?

Stage 1. Is the unit output of product or service standardized and controllable? If not, are its components controllable? Ultimately it is possible to get down to the basic elements and examine process. Corrections at that level, whether basic personnel training, steps in a procedure, or ingredients in a compound, are critical if uniform results at a more complex level are to be expected.

Stage 2. Elements in the mode of delivery to the recipient, the patient. Inappropriate transmission such as a scheduling error certainly reduces quality.

Stage 3. Are current (relative) indications for product or service use reasonable and valid? What is the scatter or distribution in a large number of applications?

Stage 4. Is each individual indication under surveillance in accord with group standards? Or do the standards fail to govern all reasons for use (that is, new procedures that bypass stage 3)?

Stage 5. If the service or product passes the criteria in stages 1 to 4, does the expected or predicted change occur or does some other consequence appear?

Stage 6. Are the expected objective changes being documented in each individual application or is "a certain number of applications" or a discreet time lapse necessary before changes are measurable?

Stage 7. Are the predicted changes associated with observable benefit (positive) or with absence of otherwise likely deterioration (negative or preventive)?

In this diverse field of medicine we may often observe that all of the quality control measures are inappropriately concentrated upon one stage to the exclusion of the others. One cannot study the end result if quality is not assured in the steps to it. The regulatory agencies say they are preparing to start at ground zero by looking

for objective evidence of indications for the service. At the moment
their quality control surveillance is focused upon two elements
peripheral to the problem: (1) Is there a physician's order for that
service? (2) Was the service performed? Buildup of facilities and
paperwork to appraise the entire gamut of quality and adequacy is
not far enough along to be effective.

Among the burdens the director must carry in his search for
quality control are the nonexpert critics of the department's activities. Although their area of involvement may not be particularly
appropriate, they respond to stimuli that are not otherwise apparent. Since their common connection is with hospital committees, you
will find them agitating about the use, abuse, or overuse of certain
modalities. One common feature of their behavior is their seizure
on one or two examples of inappropriate utilization or untoward
result with an almost emotional fixation that is unaffected by contrary evidence. Sometimes they actually do perform a useful warning function, but very noisily, when abuses are occurring. But
sometimes they do not, and the director's attempts to satisfy them
with more and more evidence serves only to keep the dispute active.

The only satisfactory way to handle such critics is to proceed,
after investigating and responding to their initial cries of alarm, as
if they no longer existed. Examine the problem objectively from as
many viewpoints as possible. Occasionally the abuse is actually occurring at another hospital but the critics choose to begin the campaign in your hospital on the assumption that you must be equally
guilty. Carry out any necessary corrective measures and inform the
friends of the department what has occurred. Otherwise, wait.
Perhaps in three, five, or ten years your critics will subside and
may even partake of the department's services. Never seek a retrac-
tion or apology; for that would only reignite the controversy.

THE CHAIN OF RESPONSIBILITY

Common to all the diverse elements of quality control
is communication. From the standpoint of communication theory it

would almost seem that enemies of clear communication had designed the hospital's system. In the usual mode Agent 1, after examining a patient, vocalizes an order. Agent 2 writes the order on a piece of paper. Agent 3 transcribes the order onto another form—hopefully correctly and in toto—and hands the form to Agent 4 for delivery to Agent 5 in the correct department. Agent 5 then directs Agent 6 to carry out the order. A subsidiary loop may be required to get Agent 6 the supplies he will need to work on the patient. Occasionally Agent 1 bypasses Agent 2 and writes the order in what may be a legible manner. So if an error arises, the question is, who in the chain of six or more is responsible. The answer is either the physician who orders or, less often, the physician who is responsible for overseeing the service. The links in between are relatively immune. (See The Personnel Function, Chapter 3.)

The director must also somehow educate primary physicians to the realities of life. When he writes an order, the person who is to carry it out does not magically appear but must be arranged for. On many occasions, M.D.'s write orders that cannot be carried out for reason of lead time required, special personnel, equipment, or the need to coordinate with some other department. That has become such a problem that the ICU had to be invented. The nurses' role is to coordinate all aspects of the patient's intensive care.

Although normally the multiple-agent system, based as it is upon the principles of specialization, operates efficiently, problems arise when agents do not comprehend what they are doing and the situation is complex. Also, the principle of redundancy in reducing transmission error is almost totally ignored. That is why the chain is restricted to three in the Intensive Care Units; closer coordination is possible, and incompatible mixtures of services do not occur. It may well be that the director of a busy department can improve performance by suitably modifying the chain. In my field, obtaining authorization for Agent 6 to take orders directly from Agent 1—bypassing 2, 3, 4, and 5—substantially improved efficiency and, more importantly, quality of product. One of the problems in multiple transcription is that part of the message may be garbled or lost. That most often occurs in connection with the intent of the order—when, how, or why something should be done in the manner desired by the physician. Therein lies the personal touch that makes otherwise impersonal departments great.

5

THE
POLITICAL
SURVIVAL
FUNCTION

THE RATIONALE

Certain requirements must be met if you are ultimately to fulfill your long-range goals as department chief. First, you must be in a position to compete for the appointment. Second, you must actually receive the appointment. Third, you must survive in the post long enough to accomplish the goals you have set for yourself. To meet those requirements, you must generate enough cooperation that your progress is not one long uphill struggle; accordingly, the requirements entail political activity. Except for the fortunate few, most physicians must engage either in conscious or unconscious political endeavors. Of course, there those whose skills are so rare and in such great demand that they can pick and choose and may be able to ignore the political exigencies until competition does appear on the horizon. In general, however, the more desirable a position is, the more competition there is for it. If there is a shortage of skilled physicians in your field, that very shortage may ultimately engender brisk competition.

As the junior associate you must please the senior department head by acting in a politically wise fashion. To maintain your relation you must behave and speak in a manner that is supportive of your superior's leadership and direction, particularly if your position depends upon his pleasure. Later, when you are in charge of the department, you will still have to play politics. A time will come when you will need $X,000 for capital acquisitions for your department. It is not likely the hospital will have many $X,000 sums to allocate, so you can be reasonably certain there will be someone else seeking the same money. Undoubtedly both you and he will have medically sound reasons for seeking the funds, so the decisions will be based as much upon politics as upon real medical necessity.

Politics is essentially a trading of advantages. To receive you must deliver, and the effectiveness of the delivery is determined by the recipient rather than by the person delivering the service. Thus your ability to survive politically is an essential attribute to your professional capacity as hospital-based physician.

OCCUPATIONAL HAZARDS

As you attain a position of eminence in the medical hierarchy, you inevitably become a potential or actual threat to someone else and others in the group may well become a threat to you. As a physician in training, you undoubtedly had reasonably good relationships with both your peers and superiors. In those special circumstances you expected and received cooperation appropriate to the situation. Consider, however, a situation in which both you and one of your peers at a hospital are eligible for a single position with incalculable professional and financial advantages. Here, obviously, you cannot expect the same quality of relationship that existed in the training situation. Each new situation alters personal relationships into forms that you may neither desire nor wish to accept.

In this context you must remember that the medical staff members who have preceded you have established and developed their political connections and so are much more influential than you. Therefore, tread cautiously through the initial stages in that organization so that you are not a real or even an implied threat to anyone's position or prerogatives. Now that will be difficult indeed if the gradient, in adequacy of training, between you and your new colleagues is steep.

A particular problem, especially for the younger specialist, is his need to watch what he says. He has just come from a situation in which freedom of expression was quite widespread. One of the reasons for that freedom was that he had no intention of staying there indefinitely. However, when you step into a situation that you hope is long-term, you need to begin to practice the art of being nice to everyone. A politically mature physician will never say anything to anyone that will cause him regret if repeated elsewhere or out of context. You must establish a reputation for being so fair and honest that even when some ill-conceived remark is attributed to you correctly, the hearer will tend not to believe you said it.

An additional hazard is the presence of what I would call the type super-A—a reference to the type A and B behavior that Dr. Friedman has so aptly described. This man is usually both talented and well-trained and is in the process of clawing his way to the top. Part of his modus operandi is to recognize and put down at the first opportunity any potential rival that he encounters. He is especially dangerous because he is so inner-directed, though he may be politically unsophisticated. Many of these super-A types later develop shortcomings and detours in their careers owing to the very intensity of their efforts and the smashing successes that in effect defeat them in their effort to reach long-term goals. However, much before the time when they themselves have been shunted onto the siding or run off the track, they tend to eliminate or seriously warp the promising careers of many innocent hospital-based physicians. These innocents may not have realized that they were in a jungle, but ignorance is no defense for either the perpetrator of the crime or his victim.

One of the advantages of joining an organization at a junior level on a salary is that a clearly dominant, politically important person is in charge. Thus, for a time, you may hide in his shadow while you study the situation. The danger is that, because your peculiar position is so safe, you may not take advantage of it to study and learn what you will need to know later. Thus when you proceed to a higher level in the hierarchy, you may be at a loss when you are forced into a confrontation that you neither anticipated nor desired. The manner in which you handle crises will in large measure determine how your career progresses. A crisis may be defined as an unanticipated problem for which you have no reasonable solution. The more innocent you are the more crises you are likely to encounter. Thus, as they say in the army, "Keep a low profile until you have thoroughly reconnoitered the situation."

HOSPITAL DIVERSITY

When Doctor X glowingly describes to you the attractive attributes of his institution, he is plainly looking at it through rose-colored glasses. He is not uncommon; most people prefer to look at only the more pleasant aspects of their situations. Whether Doctor X is unaware of the limitations of his institution or simply prefers to keep silent about them is something you will not know unless you take the time and trouble to find out. You may assume that there are negative as well as positive features in any of the offers that you receive, but dedicated work is necessary to uncover the exact nature of the negative ones.

One of the factors that makes it difficult to discern any total picture is the bewildering variety of hospitals in the United States today. A first step in making order out of this chaos is to classify the hospitals. Basically there are two major categories: those that are operated for profit and those that are not. Hospital services that are so organized that the ownership ultimately receives a profit constitute only a small fraction of the total, but they are a growing part of the U.S. scene. The reasons for their development are as varied as the motives among the population investing in the ventures. Before 1965 almost every hospital to be operated for profit was founded by an entrepreneur allied with a group of local physicians. In many instances the reasons for establishment were financial, medical, and personal. The privately owned hospitals that still retain local ownership and control are very different from those that have subsequently been taken over by corporate organizations. The importance of determining the control center of the hospital is that its location bears significantly on the speed with which decisions with financial implications can be made.

An advantage of the for-profit system is that, if some new service is both potentially valuable in terms of patient services and potentially remunerative, the ownership is likely to approve it with a minimum delay, but the delay time will vary in almost direct proportion to the number of miles between the site of the need and the site of the fiscal decision. The ethical problems of working with such a system of ownership are many, particularly if the director has an opportunity to become an investor in the hospital. Many state medical societies are taking an increasing interest in the financial relation between a physician and the hospital in which he works. Guidelines for acceptable relations are being drawn up with respect to both investment and various types of profit-sharing contracts. All those considerations must be weighed before you establish any affiliation.

The other broad group of institutions are those whose organizational needs do not require the generation of a profit from the health services delivery. This group is divisible into two major subgroups: those institutions that, to survive, must consistently break even and those that can be operated at a loss indefinitely. The first subgroup includes most of the various voluntary nonprofit hospitals such as those belonging to a church, a local community, or some school. Many of them can survive only because of substantial gifts or other income apart from that generated by their normal operating procedures. In most instances control is local, so although one can get a reasonably rapid decision about a request for funds, the problem is that often there are no funds to allocate even for a significant need.

Hospitals that are supported by taxes obviously need not be fiscally solvent. Although fiscal responsibility is desirable, these institutions provide services to a population with few resources and consequently little surplus to divert to the institution. Since services are provided for little or no return, the entire question of return on investment is not pertinent. The only question is how much of the budget can be allocated to run the institution and the department. That decision usually is made by governmental personnel who have no direct connection with the hospital's operation and who therefore see little reason to set up new services. In other institutions the incentive for setting up a new service often is that the equipment will pay for itself in the course of providing a benefit to the patients served. Since the concept of equipment paying for itself is not applicable to government-funded hospitals, the incentive for providing new services has to come entirely from other areas of pressure. Here, of course, is where politics enters the scene. Obviously, political affiliations and political ability in selling the need to get fund allocation is more valuable than in a locally controlled hospital, where the simple economics of cost recovery may be the only factor needed for a fast decision. Without political leverage, the time between request and fund allocation in a tax-supported hospital may be infinitely long.

Regulations require each health care institution to have some sort of governing board that bears ultimate responsibility for all of the activities of that institution. The kinds and complexities of governing boards are as varied as the hospitals themselves. There is no general standard except in the category of the voluntary nonprofit institution. Hospitals in the other categories—for-profit or government-supported—are in this regard a law unto themselves. The Joint Commission on Accreditation of Hospitals has outlined all of the various organizational modes that are acceptable, and the interested reader is referred to those sources.[36]

The problem of accessibility to the governing board raises the potent political question whether it is appropriate for the director to have and use such accessibility. If through chance of fortune or family or specialty the director has accessibility far beyond what he needs, he may ultimately not benefit from the access. Certainly if the medical staff or the administrator is aware of his private line to the decision makers, jealousy may reduce his gain from that resource.

If you are a relative newcomer to the scene you had best watch these activities from afar until you can sort out the most immediate factors in the environment that bear directly upon your political survival. Do not neglect studying the composition of the governing board of your hospital or of the hospitals in which you are interested. Over the long term such knowledge will prove critical to you if you are to achieve your own long-range plans.

ADMINISTRATOR DIVERSITY

Hospital administrators are as unique as any other individuals, so there is no useful system of classification except for the Theories X and Y of McGregor. As noted in a preceding section, Theory X has to do with the absolute dictator and Theory Y with the exponent of laissez faire. Although most administrators range between the two extremes in their day-to-day mode of operation, my own observation indicates that the majority are better explained by Theory X, particularly in times of crises.

Of course, the important question is not how to classify administrators in general, but how to know the particular administrator for whom you are working. As an indentured member of the medical staff, you are under far greater influence from the administrator than you might wish to be. That is unfortunate, since the programming and training of students in U.S. medical schools is toward a goal of independence in which one can operate without regard for outside opinion. If that training is coupled with your own strong independent streak, you may find severe difficulties in working as a hospital-based physician. Such an arrangement puts you in a relationship in which the differential between you and the administrator will depend far more upon the administrator's mode of action than upon your own.

If you are a very junior associate of a senior hospital-based physician, then the preceding paragraphs are really of little consequence; you are already in an obvious master-servant relationship with your immediate employer. (But you should still pay attention to the political aspects of the ongoing interrelations.) But if you are well on the way to becoming a department head, then your relationship with the administrator is of utmost importance. Owing to the very structure of the organization, his actions will have tremendous impact upon you. Therefore you must, as expeditiously as possible, get some answers about this man.

Asking blunt questions of the people you run into casually is not the way to get the information you need; in fact, those questions, repeated and transmitted, may indicate that you are in a "threatening posture" to which the administrator will react in kind. Most politically powerful and important people have a public image that they take great pains to maintain. If you go around asking questions that imply there is something else behind that facade, it will be taken as an affront. The facade almost always includes the element of being open to input from even the lowliest worker in the hospital. But unless you have some reasonable assurance that is actually the case, you had best not rely on it in making your assessment.

If the administrator is part of a highly organized hierarchial structure, such as a civil service system or a religious order, then organizationally he is an absolute dictator. Whether he utilizes all of his powers in that manner is, of course, an individual matter that must be determined. In general, however, you might assume the worst. On the other hand, if you have a voluntary, not-for-profit organization, the administrator could follow either pattern. Among the profit-making hospitals, administrators appointed by a nationwide corporation are usually merely pawns directed from higher up, but if the hospital is owned and operated locally, the administrator is likely to be someone of consequence who may follow the pattern of laissez faire (Theory Y), at least with the hospital-based physicians.

A reasonably efficacious way to identify basic policy is to find out how the last major item of capital equipment was approved. If you find that Department X suddenly turns up with a gigantic piece of costly equipment that no one else knew anything about beforehand, particularly if other departments were interested in the same function, then you may be certain that you have a Type X administrator no matter what he says. On the other hand, if you find that each piece of equipment has been brought in with the knowledge and acquiescence of most hospital departments, then the administration is Type Y. The assessment procedure, of course, is applicable only to major capital items in the multiples of thousand dollar ranges.

Another key issue is the availability of the administrator. As the department chairman, you need to have an ongoing dialogue with someone regarding what your department is doing. If you find that your dialogue is delegated to a lower-level administrative associate without decision-making powers, then that may be a sign of antagonism as well as of Type X behavior. An especially bad warning sign relative to the smooth long-term operation of the hospital and your department is a protracted wait for implementation even after you get the okay from your administrative contact, particularly about a minor matter. If all decision making stops when the administrator is not there, you have cause for alarm. A major hospital is too complex an organization to have an absentee captain, particularly an absentee Captain Queeg.

In addition to investigating major purchases, try to identify the major hospital projects and find out at what level they were initiated. If most projects were initiated by the administrator without much medical staff input, either the medical staff is grossly incompetent or the administrator is a tyrant. That is particularly true if some of the projects have little relation to the overall medical needs of the community; then it is obvious that the administrator is receiving biased information from limited sources. If you have already committed yourself in such a hospital, you have no recourse except to make the best of the situation or leave. But if you are still looking and find such a situation, take it as a good reason to look further.

It is also worthwhile to know how long the administrator has been there; a hospital with a revolving door type of administration is a disaster area. If you find that a new man has been there every year, you may be certain that the hospital has no policy except drift. There is, of course, always a chance that the next man up may be competent and able to take control. But there is also a good chance that the owners or the Board will struggle to retain absolute control even though they cannot exercise the needed day-to-day management.

Similarly important in assessing an administrator is the history of the hospital. If the hospital is fairly new, it may be that the founding member of the organization is still present as the administrator. In this case be assured that a Type X situation exists. If the hospital is that man's baby, he is going to run it in a different way than if he were a latecomer to the scene. This is not to say that a latecomer can not also be a Type X, but he will not have all the advantages of having grown up with the institution. The administrator who built and staffed the hospital is a very powerful man indeed.

The essence of all the preceding questions is whether you can enlist effective administrative support in pursuit of your goals. Many administrators are skilled in public relations and generate effusive verbal support for anyone currently in staff favor, but they never really get much done. Since they tend to respond mainly to the most overt political pressures, your chances of help are in direct proportion to your political importance. As a new or junior man at the hospital, that is not likely to be too great, so the help you can get may be minimal. If you are to be the department head or next to the department head, particularly if you are in process of establishing or improving a department's service, you undoubtedly will need space, capital funds, operational funds, and permission to increase the staff allocation.

Knowledge of just how effective the administrator is and can be in helping you get what you need is going to be invaluable to you in your assessment of the situation. There are many methods of obtaining the information you need. As a junior associate the simplest method is to ask your chief. However, for any number of reasons, he may be unable or unwilling to tell you what you need to know. In the absence of any help from the man who recruited you, you might approach one of the former chiefs of staff. That is far better than approaching the current chief for a number of political reasons. The man currently working with the administrator must perforce act as if he were on the administrator's team. If he has any sense at all, he will be most circumspect about what he says even though he may be having problems.

The ideal man to talk to is one who is several years removed from his stint as chief of staff and can safely (if he has a reasonably secure clinical practice) talk at length about the nature of the man at the top. The best time to gather such information is at a social or semisocial function, over a couple of drinks in a relaxed atmosphere. In your discussions of politics and the administrator, keep your eyes and ears open for any other information about the power structure of the hospital. Certainly, knowing the background and the present involvement of the key people in the operation of that facility is essential to the development of your political skills.

HOSPITAL POWER GROUPS

As stated, even state-run facilities must have some sort of ultimately responsible group, whether it is directors or even the legislature itself. The Board of Directors is responsible for the hospital's fiscal and goal behavior. Another level of the power structure is the chief executive officer, the administrator, who runs the hospital for the Board on a day-to-day basis. Although he is also a member of the Board, he acts as the Board's deputy. A third power is the medical staff. In government or tax-supported hospitals it may be relatively impotent. Even so, you may logically assume that there is a small coterie that wields far more influence with the decision-making levels of the hospital than the majority of the physicians. The balance of my remarks will concern hospitals whose governing boards, chief executive officer, and medical staff are active and vigorous.

The people at the top of the mountain are likely to be type A or super-A. These strong-willed people cannot coexist in easy neutrality for any length of time, since their functions tend to overlap on an almost daily basis. Their goals are not identical, and so some faction is usually trying to seize the advantage whenever an unanticipated new event changes the power balance. The basic struggle is usually between the administrator and the medical staff. They are in constant contact, and their interests are often so divergent that conflict rather than cooperation is the rule.

Even when open conflict is not present, major points of difference exist between administration and staff. Most important, perhaps, is that the administrator does not, though he may dearly wish to, control the medical staff. On the contrary, he is as much or more under their control as they are under his. That is particularly true in areas with a number of hospitals and no obvious bed shortage. Administrators who are not in full command and who are type A resent this weakness in their organizational authority and go to great lengths to get a medical executive group selected from "their men."

The governing board legally bears the ultimate responsibility for all of the activities and actions of the hospital, including those of its medical staff. The members—the trustees—are usually highly respected and wealthy persons of the business community who dedicate time, money, and effort to guiding and helping the hospital in its community service goals. They appoint and dismiss administrators; they appoint, or refuse to appoint, medical staff members; and in cases of major dispute between administration and medical staff or within the medical staff, they act as the final *ex judice* court of appeal.

However, the Board of Trustees does suffer from a serious operational weakness. Its agent, the chief executive officer, is also its prime channel of communication to and from the hospital and the medical staff. That gives the administrator a great opportunity to control and filter the flow of information, so that the Board learns only what the administrator wishes it to learn. And if in addition the administrator has a significant role in choosing who is appointed to the Board, particularly to the Board's executive committee, then his control over the Board nearly becomes ironclad. Many hospital boards and medical staffs have tried to circumvent that potential for abuse by having members of the medical staff appointed to the Board to furnish a separate line of communication. However, an astute administrator will certainly have a hand in the selection of those medical staff members; and if he has any political savvy at all, he will try to get them into his camp.

Since all of these principals are likely to have very strong egos, divergent opinions soon produce significant and serious clashes. Therefore, if there is no history or evidence of such clashes, one may be reasonably certain that the members of the group share common interests or management philosophies. Even though minor disagreements may be expressed openly, the absence of major disagreements between strong persons is prima facie evidence that they are all of the same philosophical bent.

Thus, the hospital power structure is as treacherous as an iceberg-laden sea-lane. The major portions of these monoliths lie submerged and are invisible to the casual voyager. The careers of many innocent hospital-based physicians have either foundered or been run aground by contact with one of these monoliths. However, as stormy seas make more of the iceberg visible, crises in hospitals bring out the relations between the inevitable one-up groups, provided the observer is astute enough to look for the evidence at the right time. Of course, in such a dangerous situation, it is best to observe from a safe distance. You may get a better view from closer up, but you also stand a better chance of being disastrously involved.

The type super-A medical directors who are on a fast track to the top will move into the power centers as quickly as they can in response to their own personal ego needs. But in doing so they may run a real risk of acting unwisely before they have the basic data they need to make appropriate choices. While investigating the politics of the hospital's power structure, you will lose nothing if you delay any request for alignment or alliances by pleading the press of business and your relative ignorance of the situation. That is far better than starting off by betting on the wrong horse in a building conflict; otherwise, you run a real risk of becoming a soft object between a rock and a hard place.

Once you assess the extent of power and manner of functioning of the governing board and the administrator, you should continue your study of the hospital's political situation by analyzing the medical staff's power structure. The medical staff is the most visible portion of the power iceberg; it is most likely to have an immediate effect upon you if a conflict in goals arises. If the administrator has been at the hospital for a considerable number of years, he has certainly left his mark upon the key medical staff officers. Those powerful allies of the administration may or may not be apparent to the new staff member, since they may not necessarily occupy key power positions at the moment. Therefore, it is essential to move cautiously while you try to identify them.

A rational though rarely taken approach to this problem is to thoroughly read and study a document that every new staff member receives, the hospital's medical staff bylaws. As required by the Joint Commission, the bylaws outline in detail the medical staff structure and function, particularly the actions that must be taken in the selection of the chairmen of the key committees and the other members of the medical Executive Committee. Therefore, instead of immediately placing the bylaws in the nearest round file—the almost universal practice—the budding medical director should study the document very carefully. It will provide him with some immediate answers regarding who does what, as for example, whether the Committee chairmen are appointed by the chief of staff or are elected by the Committee membership. If they are appointed, you have a single target on which to concentrate your wiles should you wish to be a contender. If they are elected, you need to do a lot more politicking on the broader level among the Committee membership.

The bylaws will also describe how the nominating committee is constituted. That will not only tell you how the power group perpetuates itself but may also indicate a way in which you can prepare to insinuate yourself into that group. Further, there will be some indication in the bylaws of the goal and philosophy of the hospital. Of course, much of the operational philosophy will remain unwritten. Additionally, it may be that the bylaws are merely a copy of the model bylaws recommended by the Joint Commission.

If the hospital has been in existence for a number of years, however, it is very likely that the document will gradually develop a subtle flavor evolving from that hospital's ideals, goals, and service orientation. Obviously, that will not be detectable at a single casual reading; it may require some study and thought and research.

I have observed that even in government departments there can be major differences in philosophy that remain unstated. There are government departments in which the philosophy is that "everything that is not expressly forbidden is thereby permitted." And there are other departments in which "all that is not expressly permitted is thereby forbidden." These are important matters that must be deduced by the director; for they will certainly determine his degree of freedom in reacting to the demands upon himself and his department. That is not insignificant. We have already seen that a director may respond to a perceived need in a manner that will raise a threat among other departments because the action is out of keeping with the overall approach of the institution.

THE BASIC PHILOSOPHY OF THE HOSPITAL

In fairness to new staff members, it would be ideal if the power group of the hospital had inscribed upon a brass plaque the hospital's basic philosophy. Even when the hospital does try to document its philosophy, however, the words often bear no accurate relation to what actually occurs. If the institution were offered five types of needed services, its choices in order of priority would be determined by its actual operational philosophies, and not by the words in its bylaws. All too often by the time the director realizes that his goals and those of the institution are dissimilar, he has committed himself to working in that area and in that hospital. As is usually the case, the lesser part does most of the accommodating in cases of discrepancy.

A particularly disturbing approach is a peculiar mix of laissez faire combined with dictatorship (Type X): the administrator acts dictatorially in general but grants a limited laissez faire capability to certain specific department chairmen in their own spheres of interest. The departments are sensitive not to community need or medical staff interests, but rather to the financial and practical needs of their chairmen. In essence the hospital, or a portion of it, is being run for the personal convenience of key staff men. The clinically oriented medical director can hardly expect his own aims to be compatible with that which is personally convenient for the people in power. Conflict is inevitable; the only question is how soon and under what terms.

The selection process insures that like-minded persons will be chosen for the positions of power. It would be interesting to collect data on the number of medical staff who have never been on a committee at certain institutions and on the repetitive assignments of a smaller, more select group. Occasionally a maverick slips in and becomes a prominent officeholder, but in most instances a holding action develops among the in group during his tenure so that his appointment has little effect. The long-range strength of such power groups is that it is so pervasive that it eventually discourages unlike-minded physicians from staying in that area. A key question to ask various junior members of the staff, accordingly, is whether they are comfortable working in the place. If several answer no, particularly if they have membership among several hospitals and so can compare, take heed. Of course if you happen to be in total accord with the philosophy of the power group, then you probably will not encounter conflict and undoubtedly you will prosper.

From all the foregoing you can see that if you make a bad alliance or act contrary to the hospital's philosophy, you will be in trouble. The worst mistake, however, is not the bad alliances (since you can always disavow them on the grounds of ignorance) but being marked as a person who does not "see things the way they are." There is nothing wrong with "right thinking" provided it does not insist upon an absolute monopoly. Certainly the greatest progress is made by institutions all of whose members face in the same direction at the same time and move forward in step. What is not conducive to progress is intolerance to the point of actual active harassment of other approaches to a problem.

Every department head needs enough political clout to get certain things done, such as acquiring new equipment, new service, new staff, or new space. To obtain the concrete wherewithal, it is important that you not cut yourself off from the inner councils. It is essential to interract with as many of the medical staff as you can on a positive level or, failing that, on as neutral a level as possible. You need to have multiple daily contact with your peers. In that way you can identify the key people to talk to whenever important decisions are at hand, and you can set up a system that enables you to get to those people in short order and in a manner most conducive to making your case.

To do your job properly, therefore, you must approach each member of the medical staff with the attitude that "it really costs me nothing to be nice to this man, but it sure as hell may cost me later if I am not." All of this is a rather calculating type of approach, but it has the merit of a high survival value. Being a smart aleck is no way to build up a power base; it is a good way to erode whatever power accompanies the position to which you were appointed.

COMMITTEES

The easiest way to destroy a hospital-based physician is to continually chip away at his requests in committees by delaying or sidetracking them for procedural reasons. Each delaying action is so minor that it is soon forgotten, except by the target of the action, but it has a cumulative effect. After a while everyone will be saying, "God, he really isn't very effective, is he?" If you are to develop a reputation for effectiveness and success, it is imperative that the majority of your committee requests be granted. In addition, your successes must be highly visible to build up your reputation and increase your input into the power circles.

The committee is the organizational unit of the hospital's medical staff structure. Its function is to receive input from a variety of members who then work out jointly accepted policies and develop plans appropriate for the long-term pull. Although the implementation of those plans may be the prerogative of single individuals, development of and agreement on the plans inevitably requires group action. A more thorough enumeration of the functions of committees would include the following:

—To mutually educate the membership in the complexities of a given situation.

—To develop a consensus on an agreeable response in a complex situation.

—When alternative actions are possible, to choose the best one.

—To provide a meeting ground, with formal rules of conduct, for resolution of actual or potential conflicts among opposing points of view.

—To provide a forum for planning with additional input from less concerned areas.

—To coordinate the actions of one or more groups.

—To provide a formal setting for peer review or other judicial processes.

—To formally and openly review the qualifications of new applicants to the staff.

—To provide an effective means of communication with another organization, particularly one at a higher level. (In general, rigidly structured groups have great difficulty in communicating with an individual except insofar as he is a representative of another group. Therefore, if you wish to communicate with an organized group, especially at government level, it is best to invest your input with the same trappings.)

Unless you have a direct line to the power center of the hospital, each of your proposed activities and requests must go through one committee or another on its way to the decision-making level. Even in the event you feel that the committee structure is a farce as presently constituted, you must proceed in the proper manner, for everyone will expect that approach. If you manage the presentation adequately and do not run into obstructionists, you may actually generate a useful degree of support.

The traditional departments—Radiology, Pathology, and

Anesthesiology—may or may not have specific departmental committees, but they invariably have one important asset: the heads of
their departments sit on the Executive Committee. The chief
pathologist, radiologist, and anesthesiologist may not have votes on
that Committee, but their very presence gives them an additional
power connection that other department heads do not have. If your
specialty and your position grant you admission to that select circle, then you are well on your way to achieving your departmental
goals.

As the new head of a department you may be offered the
chairmanship of a subcommittee relating to your department's activities. Before you accept the offer, it is wise to find out a few
details. If you accept, will you have any other committee appointments or will you remain in a cul-de-sac? If you do have the opportunity to be on a major committee as well, then this subcommittee
may be of little use to you. Its disadvantage is that it must answer
to a parent committee; another level is interposed between you and
the decision-making Executive Committee. Every matter must be
voted upon not only in your subcommittee but again in the parent
committee before going to the Executive Committee—three opportunities for harassment or derailment. In an urgent situation the
very time delay in getting the parent committee to approve your
resolution may effectively obstruct appropriate action. Additionally, if there is any real financial or legal implication to your action,
it must go to the hospital's Board of Governors, a step that guaran-
tees still further delays.

It is also important to know whether you will be chairman of
that subcommittee. If so, will the membership be chosen by you or
by the chief of staff? The chief of staff, if not neutral, could easily
put people on that subcommittee who could thoroughly impede
your work. You might be better off to take your business to where
your main strength lies. The major new departmental specialties
fall mainly under the Department of Medicine (Cardiology, Respiratory Services, Neurology, Nephrology, Nuclear Medicine,
Hematology, and so on). You may be better off being in a group

situation with the prime consumers of your services. There you will have a ready forum for practical therapeutic suggestions from the people who utilize the product and you will have regularly scheduled meetings with the consumers of your product with interchange and feedback.

A list of the regular hospital medical staff committees includes:

Executive Committee of the Medical Staff
Joint Conference Committee—Executive Committee and Hospital Board representation
Department of Medicine
Department of Surgery
Department of Family Practice
Department of Pediatrics
Department of Obstetrics and Gynecology
Department of Anesthesia
Department of Outpatient Services and Emergency Room
Department of Radiology
Department of Pathology and Laboratory Services
Tissue and Transfusion Committee
Utilization Review Committee
Credentials Committee
Critical Care Committee
Infectious Diseases Committee
Continuing Medical Education Committee
Patient Care Services Committee
Medical Records Committee
Library Committee
Pharmacy Committee
Medical Care Evaluation or Audit and Peer Review Committee

In addition, many subspecialty departments, both medical and surgical, have their own subcommittees. Obviously, with this choice array you will have the opportunity for one or more committee appointments, but you must make sure you get an appointment that satisfies your primary commitments. Those commitments, of course, are determined by whoever pays the major portion of your income. Hopefully there will be no conflict between the services you are expected to perform for the hospital and the duties that accompany your committee assignments.

The advantage of multiple committee assignments is the opportunity to choose the most suitable location for expounding new proposals and ideas. The disadvantage is that if your department is involved in more than one committee and you cannot be present at all of the meetings, you may be assured, by the principle of Murphy's law, that if something can go wrong, it will. It is in the one meeting you miss that your department will be discussed in far greater detail than you might have wished. Of course, that can also happen on committees of which you are not a member. If you have a structured department with a departmental supervisor appointed by the hospital, it is useful to make his availability known to all committee chairmen. Thus if questions arise and you are not available to answer them, the questioners can at least get the supervisor.

You may also request that the supervisor be allowed to attend meetings when you are not available, not only to provide necessary departmental input but also to receive feedback that might modify departmental activities. Unfortunately, physicians on the whole prefer not to have nonphysicians at their meetings, owing to the delicate matters that they sometimes discuss in a rather spontaneous fashion. It is increasingly common for administrative personnel to be present at major committee meetings, but it would be politick to get approval before you have your assistant stand in for you.

A further disadvantage to multiple committee assignments derives from the antagonism of practicing physicians toward hospital-based physicians. The cause of this antagonism associated with committees is that the clinical members are not paid for their time in committee whereas the hospital-based physician is assumed to be paid whether he attends or not. The practicing physicians therefore tend to be vehement in their comments about the absence of physicians who are on salary or retainer from the hospital. If you must absent yourself, it is wise to have another committee member aware of your good reasons for nonattendance. Hopefully he will relay that information if comments are made about your absence. If you are absent because you are golfing, you may hope that no one will volunteer any information at all.

Professional antagonism is apparent not only in committees but in other areas as well. It is extraordinary how many physicians can know whether a particular hospital-based physician is present by looking around the parking lot. A tendency at a number of hospitals is for prominent physicians, particularly those who are not the director's fans, to drop by the department on one pretext or another to see the director; it becomes obvious, from the frequency of the visits and from feigned astonishment at the director's absence, that their real purpose is to see if he is putting in his time. Obviously if your contractual obligation requires you to be in your department at specified times, you had best be there over the major portion of the year. However, if your contractual obligations have no time stipulations, you may have to satisfy curious gentlemen by having the departmental secretary offer to get you on the phone immediately.

There are a number of other problems with committees. First, the physician man-hour cost of most decisions is rather exorbitant. If relations of trust prevailed among the committee members, far more committee work could be delegated to work groups and rubberstamped by the parent committee. In connection with complex matters, most committees provide advance background information about the issues to be discussed. However, that information is almost uniformly ignored by the committee members, so that tremendous amounts of time must be wasted while the members are being educated on the background detail. That lack of preparation displays the very essence of arrogance—"a condition in which an excess of ego is compounded by an equal excess of ignorance."

A second problem is that the larger and more complex the group the more decisions must be watered down to gain general approval. In the words of Dr. Norman Koenig, "Conscience gets a lot of credit for what is actually a case of cold feet." Third, if there is a dominant member at the meeting, the entire committee time may be wasted, since only the one man's viewpoints will be broadcast and acted upon. It is exceedingly wasteful to spend five or six physician man-hours to rubberstamp one man's decision. Finally, committees are convenient forums for passing the buck by means of tabling an action or sending it back to a subcommittee or working group for further study. The politically astute often use that ploy to harass their rivals in the hospital.

COMMUNICATION SKILLS

As we discussed previously, the administrator is in a key position to receive information from throughout the hospital. If he chooses, he can pass along only the portions that are supportive of his position. From that point of view you can see that an adequate command position in the communication network is vital if you are to be effective in any hospital environment. In fact, a major function of the director of a department is to be fully aware of what is going on in the department itself, as well as its interactions with all the other departments in the hospital. That is a function no one except the physician can effectively perform, since a lesser trained person cannot fully appreciate all of the various levels of interaction between areas. You must build up an information-gathering network that is effective, selective, and reliable and that provides you with useful information.

If you wish to learn as expeditiously as possible, the technique is to listen, not talk. That may seem to be a trite observation, but it is as commonly ignored by physicians as it is accurate. Even in a matter of conflict it is advantageous to listen; for your opponent may inadvertently reveal facts and feelings that will strengthen your position. In conversations with others, observe whether you are merely waiting to spring into verbal action or really paying attention to what the other person is saying. A crucial part of your political survival depends upon the rapid acquisition of correct information. Particularly when you are working from a small power base, you need to have all the information you can get. Your intense concentration upon what the other person is saying will at least leave him with a more favorable impression.

With the exception of a few who have ongoing daily commitments, physicians spend a small portion of their total time in the hospital. Therefore, their period of observation and the volume of information they receive is limited. The nonmedical personnel of the hospital, on the other hand, spend forty hours there each week. Accordingly, they are more likely than you to see and hear about many events that may be of particular interest to you. Five nurses in the ICU will probably provide you with far more information about what is going on there than will five doctors who have patients in it.

Hopefully you will give the input from nonmedical personnel the respect it deserves. It is not uncommon for someone to call the doctor with important information and receive a tongue-lashing for disturbing him. If you emulate that ancient custom of cutting off the head of the bearer of bad tidings, you will soon not hear anything troublesome, whether it is important to you or not. On numerous occasions I have seen groups of nurses, in intensive care units at night, agonizing over which one will draw the short straw and have to call Doctor X. Something has gone wrong with Doctor X's patient that he should know about. But instead of calling Doctor X immediately, they delay for reason of a certain tongue-lashing.

In spite of its stupidity, that behavior is commonplace in countless hospitals. The ideal way to receive information is to maintain an open and cordial relationship with every staff member with whom you have regular contact. Know the members by their faces if not their names and be cheerful and positive with them. Undoubtedly you will receive more information than you really need, but it is only you who can decide that. A moment's reflection is sufficient to realize that if a nurse knew as much as you and could decide what you needed to know, she would no longer be a nurse, she would be a doctor, and she would be working for herself, not for you. Therefore, there is no reason to be irritated if someone gives you unnecessary information; only you can know if you need it or not. Since most people have many more things to do than go out of their way to deliver information to you, your greatest fear should be that you get too little information rather than too much.

DELIVERY OF INFORMATION

Information, like water, flows best downhill; uphill flow requires external pressure. In the case of information, the gradient is in the mind of the recipient. Thus, to get information to one of your colleagues you may have to transpose it to a level sufficiently high that he will accept it without opposition or question (from a visiting expert?). Information you transmit to lower-echelon personnel will automatically be heard and accepted; in fact, this is one way to get facts to your peers. Suppose you wish them to do process A and toward that end you have a visiting expert talking about process A. That will no doubt do some good, but you will get even better compliance if you can get the same message across to the hospital's nursing staff so that they can appropriately remind the doctors about process A. Since they heard about it from Professor X, it must be okay and the reinforcement is accepted.

That procedure will work only if you have taken the time and trouble to get the information delivered from the top—the visiting expert—as well as from below. Ordinarily, attempting to get information to the doctor from below is a wasted effort except in special circumstances in which the physician clearly is out of his depth and will rely upon advice from nonmedical personnel. In most instances doctors solicit help by asking what Doctor Z would do in this case; they then write down the order "Follow Doctor Z's protocol." Here the hospital personnel can be useful by identifying the puzzled doctor. When word gets back to the director, he can take action by organizing a learning situation that will reach the physician.

If you approach communication from the same standpoint as you approach the diagnosis of a difficult case, you will probably have less trouble. When you encounter a complex illness, your first step is to accumulate an adequate data base. Until you have acquired the data base, you do not propose or initiate long-range solutions; you confine your action to short-range ones that an emergency situation may require. You listen, examine, question, requestion, and reexamine until finally you have a reasonable hypothesis that you test against the facts of the situation; only at that point do you begin the appropriate long-term therapy.

Similarly, when there is a major problem in the hospital, you must first acquire the adequate data base. At no time do you respond without information unless the situation is so clearly delineated that further search is unnecessary. While it may be salutory to your ego to make a snap decision on the basis of a similar situation you have seen before, it is highly unlikely that the two situations are exactly identical, so a snap decision may not be altogether appropriate.

If you are the associate of or assistant to a senior man, you had best establish the most cordial of relationships with him in order to receive all of his input and advice. Of course, the information he gives will no longer be entirely relevant because the situation will no doubt have changed, but the background detail can be of immense importance to you in forging the best patterns of development in your own response. Soliciting information from an older man may be difficult for some of the younger subspecialists who feel that their ability to perform a multitude of highly specialized procedures makes them experts in all stages of medical care and politics. However, throughout the nation, particularly in government and industry, the common denominator among people chosen for the top leadership is the breadth of their experience, interest, talents, and abilities, and not the presence of special technical skills. Leaders are not selected on the basis of special skills except perhaps that talent or trick of getting elected.

A top leader pulls in the personnel with the special skills he needs at appropriate times. Each medical director ought to do likewise. Therefore, if you do not have all of the experience you need, you can obtain surrogate experience by questioning others who have been that way before. Again, you must listen, not talk or editorialize. It will take you some time to gather information that

way, but it would take you considerably more time to individually experience and react to all the instances you are hearing about.

YOUR POWER BASE

The best power base a doctor can have is a superlatively
working department that meshes with all other hospital functions.
In that one area, no one can challenge him. Those who are unable
to reach his level of output may feel acutely threatened by it, but
they will find it hard to complain about. It may even precipitate an
abnormal psychological reaction in others, specifically the use of
projection. The empire builders will accuse you, because of your
very success, of empire building. Your only consolation is that appropriate delivery of relevant services to the consumer at a reasonable price is the criterion of success and that the others are welcome to join you at that level.

The second step in developing your power base is to convert
your department employees into missionaries who let it be known
how effective they are as a team. This should not be an idolatory
type of evangelism designed merely to bolster your ego; instead it
should be a team spirit whose message is that results are due to the
team and not to a hero. If each of your staff does public relations
work for the department, you will have a much more stable political base.

The third step in developing your power base is to enroll in the
hospital's in-service training program. There is always a shortage of
talent to speak to the other departments who need some educational enrichment. If you gain the reputation of being open and
agreeable to educating, not only will you have more requests for
talks and lectures in the hospital but additional people will spread
your reputation and that of your department throughout the community. Moreover, those people will be able to integrate better
with your department personnel and so indirectly will improve
your department's performance. Ultimately, you may even extend
your influence into the community—by word-of-mouth reputation
and without becoming involved in the community activities.

Many people in medicine either are born with or develop a flair for showmanship. Used correctly, showmanship can enhance your own and your department's reputation for a very good reason: a showman keeps proving his point, that is, his excellence. Your act consists of continually providing competent care and superior services on a daily basis. Thus showmanship must be sustained, since the people who arrive on your doorstep will come with higher than normal expectations. It would be disastrous if you became unable to provide the clinical help that earlier gave you your wide reputation. Arguments and explanations of why you cannot deliver the product today or this year will simply not be satisfactory. Both patients and staff physicians have a very poor loyalty index, and in the event of disappointment they will go from a positive to a negative attitude very quickly.

In the same vein, if you are a clinical specialist, effective management carries another hazard. The more time you devote to management, the more likely you are to lose touch with some of the basic medical techniques that you once performed yourself. That is especially apt to happen if you are the manager of a large department with a considerable number of other physicians who perform the services that you once performed so well yourself. After a prolonged period of handling other people and delegating most of the work, you may suddenly find yourself challenged by an associate on the basis of your decreased technical competence. What the challenger fails to realize is that, as manager, you have a far broader viewpoint of all the interrelations in that service, and that, theoretically, should make up for your rustiness in technical matters. What you may not realize, however, is that most staff physicians will not give you any theoretical credit for your expertise in management in view of your rustiness in medicine. To be treated as a doctor, you must continue doctoring. All that creates additional pressures on you to perform at a higher level than before, because you have got to learn the new while keeping up with the old. Otherwise, you may lose some or even all of the power base you are building.

Once you develop a solid foundation of support within the department, the hospital, and the medical staff, you might consider auxiliary or alternative power bases. One such base, if the option is open to you, is development of an outside source of income, possibly another hospital department, a limited office practice or laboratory, or a contract for services with an outside group of physicians. That would provide insurance if a major confrontation due to a change in administration or politics were to occur and your contract was terminated. Otherwise, you would have to file for bankruptcy.

The particular kind of alternative base you choose will, of course, depend upon your options and needs. You may have a perfectly satisfactory relation with the administrator and the power structure of the hospital at this moment. Consequently, you may feel no need to take any precautions, or there may be no obvious option for such an action on your part. However, all humans and human relations are mortal, and the man with whom you have established such an excellent relationship may suddenly not be there anymore. You may find that the rules of the game have changed because the players have been changed. That is probably the most potent reason for medical directors looking to have other strings to their bows.

Another power base also gives you the option of adding more help to the position by generating the financial wherewithal. You may have had offers to affiliate with a group in primary practice, or to accept a salaried position at a tax-supported hospital, or to acquire another medical directorship at a nearby hospital. The last alternative is potentially the most attractive provided that, in case of serious conflict of interests, both administrators do not act in concert to cut you off simultaneously. In one instance a medical director became grossly inadequate in his performance at two hospitals he was servicing, and the two administrations joined forces in efforts to remove him in that same year. He had no alternative but to leave the area and to go elsewhere.

The danger in developing an alternative power base is the possibility that it will distract you from your primary function. Feedback from the people to whom you are providing services will permit you to judge whether that service continues to be adequate. But make sure that the feedback you solicit comes from people who have no reason to lie to you. If you ask your wife or your chief supervisor or your secretary if you are doing okay, the price of saying anything other than what you want to hear may be more than he or she wishes to pay. Even the administrator may assure you that everything is all right until some critical issue occurs and he decides to lower the boom.

The more diverse your activities, the more diverse must be your sources of information. It would be delightful if you could rely upon the medical staff to tell you when you are not providing what they want. However, most people won't bother complaining until the problems become major. If your first warning of a problem is a major complaint, it may be too late because it may be followed by an avalanche of major complaints all of the same nature. Thus you must demand more from your doctors; more than the simple assurance that you are doing okay, you should expect an adequate critique. In short, the absence of complaints is insufficient assurance that your alternative power base is not interfering with your prime function. If you become incautious, you may find that, in your attempt to increase your power base, you have amputated a major portion of it.

THE INDEPENDENT PERSPECTIVE

The subject of this chapter is not necessarily pleasant. Physicians are trained to work with patients, provide care, and keep on doing the same. Political activities have little to do with that primary function, even though they are essential to your continuing to operate as a physician. Whether you enjoy the political aspects of your profession or not, it is important to avoid being driven into a corner emotionally or mentally and reacting in ways that are not appropriate. Thus, in addition to having an alternative power base, you must also have access to a different kind of world than the one in which you are immersed.

I would recommend that you try to keep a major portion of

your personal life separate from your professional activities. If your only relief from work is mingling and meeting with the same people you see every day at the hospital, you really cannot escape the situation. That means you should develop social relations with other people than those with whom you work. Perhaps you can rely upon your wife for contact in other areas if you do not have primary contact yourself. You need the contact to maintain a sense of how other people work and live and think and also to provide an opportunity to let your hair down someplace from which tales about what you said when you had one too many will not be carried back.

Additionally, it is essential that you avoid one of the pitfalls of an incestuous medical relationship: the interpersonal conflicts that occasionally arise among a few wives of members of the hospital medical staff. Sometimes a small group of the women involved develop strong feelings because of the private input they receive from their husbands. Any public display of their likes and dislikes can alter what might otherwise have been a satisfactory working relationship. This is most apt to happen when your wife's only social contact is with the wives of the physicians with whom you are working. But some doctors' wives can be even more prickly about their prerogatives and their status than the doctors themselves. If both of you are on stage every moment you are in a social relation, the strain may become too great and events that are not conducive to meeting your long-term goals may occur.

6
FINDING YOUR NICHE

DEFINING YOUR TARGET

The prospective medical director must mount a long-range, full-scale campaign if he wishes to find a post that will approximate his ultimate requirements. It is amusing to note that, regardless of specialty, the majority of departmental directors discount chance and luck as significant determinants of their present positions. They pat themselves on the back for the series of decisions that led to their current situations, but they remain unable to give any useful information about how to attain an equivalent post. The simple remark most consistently made is that "You have to be in the right spot at the right time." This obviously is of little or no help to anyone who does not know where the right spot is and when the right time is. But by being aware of how vulnerable you are to fortuitous events, you may take far more care in planning all of the actions that are within control.

This chapter is concerned with preparing for and conducting a campaign to find a desired position, determining the various levels of opportunities in each potential position, recognizing the implicit contract you establish with the medical staff upon assumption of a directorship, and identifying some of the pitfalls awaiting the un-wary. The first consideration in determining your ultimate goal is your choice of specialty; obviously, that choice will limit the nature and variety of your options. If your goal is to be director, no mat-ter what the specialty, you will do well to pick an area noted for scarcity of talent but in great demand—or be prepared to move into a geographical area with less competition.

Since there is no overall shortage of qualified candidates in the traditional fields of pathology, radiology, and anesthesiology, there are few attractive posts currently vacant in those areas; whatever vacancies occur are so ephemeral that, unless you are already in position the moment the opening occurs, you will never have a chance. It is sometimes possible to make the chance for yourself by finding a group that is about to establish a new hospital and allying yourself with it financially or otherwise so you are the obvious choice for a department head. Otherwise, you must be prepared to spend a good deal of time as either an assistant or an associate to a medical director.

Here, of course, is where the vagaries of fate—illness of doctor or in his family, catastrophe, retirement, death—may put you into position as a prime contender when a vacancy does occur. From that point of view, to achieve your goal quickly you should look for a position with an older man whose working expectancy might be limited. However, be aware that most physicians, by selection pressure, tend to be very long-lived, and so yours may not be a short wait. Additionally, rigidity of behavior often accompanies in-creasing age, so you may have more than normal difficulty in work-ing closely with such a person—particularly if you hope to estab-lish a relationship such that he would recommend you as his suc-cessor.

The young physician should realize that in the nonclinical areas, particularly in pathology and radiology, some older estab-lished directors tend to exploit the younger specialists by hiring them on a revolving door basis. These more powerful members of the fraternity use the societies' employment agencies to assure themselves of adequate help that will never threaten their positions.

They take on young politically naive physicians at a fixed salary commitment for several years; and by the time the assistant expects to advance in remuneration and responsibility, he suddenly finds his services terminated and a new junior assistant replacing him. Of course, such a position may be your only alternative until you acquire sufficient experience, maturity, and financial stability to strike out on your own.

In the meantime, learn as much as possible about the politics and the fine machinations involved in dealing with one key older man. By not putting yourself out on a limb by ignoring the inevitable, you may actually enlist the help of such an older person in getting you something more suitable later on. You may also begin to develop the knack of establishing your own staff loyalties—loyalties that will be useful to you in future years—rather than the haphazard type of friendships that most persons tend to establish. Because of the contacts you have made and the help (or at least lack of opposition) that you have engendered, you may be able to leave the scene for something better at your convenience rather than at the convenience of your employer.

If you are the nth person in an n-man group, you are not in direct line for succession when the leader departs the scene. Your ascent to a more primary role will depend upon how you conduct yourself in the group setting. To climb, seize every opportunity and devote the time required to master the administrative work that the group needs done—scheduling, conferring with office manager and personnel, riding herd on the various benefits, plans, and insurance, and so forth. In the words of Dr. Neal Hamel, "You will find that he who administers—ultimately directs." That may indeed be your shortcut to the top, since everyone else is too busy doctoring to learn the ABC's of management at that practical level.

On the other hand, you may have wisely allowed for a period in a subsidiary role to gain additional experience and insight. Although you may be very well trained and the only experience you seek to acquire is that of learning to manipulate and work with and around people, your added specialty experience will still be a plus factor. The greater the competition among your peers, the more you need to gain assets that set you above and apart from your competitors. One such way is to stay on at your training institution in a different role, no longer a trainee. Your strategy should be to use the position to develop wide contacts in addition to acquiring additional experience.

In clinical fields (cardiology, neurology, gastroenterology, respiratory, nephrology) the supply of talent relative to demand ranges from a buyer's to a seller's market. However, most physicians with the qualifications to become medical directors, when faced with a lack of immediate opportunity, tend to drift into direct patient care activities as a prompt means of achieving financial solvency. They thereby remove themselves from the scene as active competitors for positions that arise subsequently. If one of them does try to attain the position of director, he will usually need to recruit a young associate to give him the time and professional resources to handle both tasks. In that way you may come upon several indirect opportunities—indirect since they require affiliating with someone in practice and acting as his deputy in running the department.

The flight to the suburbs among middle- and upper-class Americans obviously affects the extent of such opportunities. If you are prepared to go into the smaller towns and rural areas, you are likely to find no one competing for such minor positions as exist. The same thing may be true if you are prepared to go into the inner core of the larger cities; for there the volume is great enough to insure the existence of such openings. The intermediate area is likely to be the one that is in greatest demand. Thus one way you must define your target is by listing the limitations upon its locus. Not everyone can live and practice in Hawaii. Restricting your choice to areas celebrated for their beneficial climates or their recreational advantages is unwise, particularly if you expect to attain the upper level of income in your specialty.

The more intense the competition the more the price will be bid down. A case in point is the desirability of San Francisco as a practice locus for a physician. If a doctor moves into that area as either

an associate or an independent practitioner, he should be prepared to earn substantially less than he could anywhere else in California. Since San Francisco's cost of living is not lower than elsewhere, that implies sacrificing a considerable amount of money for
the privilege of living in a particular area. If the area is vital, so be
it. Most physicians, however, have other interests than the mean
temperature, so the dispersion of talent around the country is still
reasonably meshed with the demand for services. But if you are
going to restrict your search for a position to a highly desirable,
and hence competitive, area, you must be prepared to do far more
preparatory work before you find your permanent niche.

FINDING YOUR TARGET

Once you have defined what you are willing to do and
where you are willing to do it, you must home in on a specific
target. The most satisfactory placements are usually made through
personal contacts; it is insufficient to make contact only through
the mails or by weekend visits. If it is at all feasible, it is best to
spend the last years of your training in institutions in the area in
which you are interested. If you cannot do your last year of training in your preferred area, then you should assign one or more
years to working, after training is completed, in that area, in order
to gain the personal contacts that you need.

If that is to be your approach, it may be best to seek a position
in a large medical group or hospital so as to maintain as low a
profile as possible. As only a cog in the machinery, you will have
definite hours on and hence, more importantly, definite hours off
to pursue your investigation and research. Large groups have the
additional advantage of fostering more than the usual amount of
professional traffic, which increases your opportunities to make
contacts.

Finding such a position is not really difficult if you are persistent and begin the search well in advance of need. The resources
are the classified sections in the medical journals and throwaways
and the job employment services (if they exist) of the professional

societies. While delightful to think about, the chances of answering an ad from a thousand miles away and being accepted and ensconced in a delightful lifelong relationship is so remote as to not warrant any effort of consideration. What you should be expecting to find is a short-term position from which to launch your search for the opportunity that will satisfy your long-term objectives. Thus the post should be in the mainstream of medical activity in the area to give you the strategic perspective you will need.

Each and every special field in medicine has its own society, and each society maintains a roster of members arranged geographically. Thus a task worthy of at least a few hours activity, once you are in the search area, is to list all the members of your specialty in the area and then search out the biographical details of each in the directories of the American Medical Association and the various major specialties. Then you should scout around among the members of the medical profession whom you personally know until you find someone who knows them. The details you gain may be of use in plotting further action. Unless clearly contraindicated, call them, introduce yourself, and ask for advice as a newcomer in the area.

A word of caution about a common technique designed to limit your options at the earliest possible moment. Certain large groups dominant in an area may encourage their newest junior associate to invest immediately, usually in a personal residence, in the expectation that he will then be committed to that area and hence to them. Unless you have a ready facility for handling real estate purchases and sales, you should avoid such early commitments, since they may prove an embarrassing drag to you in your long-range plans. A related technique is to tie you down by means of social commitments. Country club memberships and other such entanglements are a cheaper way of keeping you than paying you more money or giving you more responsibility. Therefore, be suspicious of any bargains involving deals that would tie you down financially far sooner than you had planned.

Your chief strength during this entire incubation period will be your frame of mind. If you are prepared to learn from your own and others' mistakes and not to assume that you are indeed the captain of your ship, you may find this transitional period very valuable. But that is possible only if you are aware of the controllable and uncontrollable aspects of the decisions that you make. At one time it was a sign of character weakness to move more often than once every five years. Today it is well recognized that sometimes all that is to be learned in a particular area can be learned in a year and that those who stay longer than that are foolish or immature. Thus you should be ready to move when it is best for your long-term career, provided you satisfy whatever obligations you have undertaken.

It is foolish to move for only a possibly better option if in so doing you develop a reputation for untrustworthiness. Such a reputation can spread faster than you can travel, and it may give you trouble in the future. The network of personal interrelation in the medical community is so intricate that you may not be aware of a significant channel of communication between people in two apparently disparate areas. Quite obviously, if you are working for someone under an obligation and you are presented with a valuable but short-lived opportunity, your superior may release you. However, in most instances such considerations are in the mind of the person who wishes to leave rather than in the facts of the situation, so in effect you are being released because you are immature enough to fall for self-deception.

SPECIFIC SUGGESTIONS

With the above generalities established we can begin looking at more specific suggestions. If you are going through a period of association or preceptorship, try to extract from that situation as much experience as possible. Undoubtedly the senior department head will use your talents to his own purpose, but hopefully you can establish a relationship with him such that ultimately he will help you rather than merely discard you because you have become either too expensive or too threatening. Be open and frank with him about the transitory nature of your position and its usefulness to you in your career plan. You may be able to enlist his help in moving you out on your terms as well as his.

One of the advantages of joining a group in the area in which you hope eventually to locate is the opportunity to remain without political affiliations. Thus you have time to study the situation and identify the most advantageous alliances and contacts. As a new member in the area, the danger of your making a politically disadvantageous alliance is relatively remote. But it is not totally absent, and there are unscrupulous physicians who are only too willing to subvert your good-natured intentions to their own desires. By clearly making you their man, they may make you unacceptable to anyone else in that community. You will then have no alternative but to work with that group or leave.

In Chapter 7 we shall raise the problem of the senior man in effect "importing and subsidizing his competition." That, of course, is an option open to you if you are affiliated with someone with whom you clearly cannot work in harness for long: you stay just long enough to learn your senior's weaknesses and then move out and set up a competing shop. That is not likely to get you the directorship of any institution in which your senior is more influential than you are, but it may well be that his political career is in the declining phase. If you are wise and lucky enough, you may be able to take a shortcut to your ultimate goal. It is easier, however, to leave a group association without generating negative feelings—even though you are staying in the community and setting up an effective competition—than it is to leave a single person. Almost invariably when a senior physician takes in a junior associate who subsequently separates and sets up his own practice, the parting generates considerable acrimony and political infighting.

That is really not too important to a practicing physician whose long-term survival depends mainly upon his acceptance by a large group of patients. But if your plan is to eschew private practice in favor of a hospital-based position, such a controversy will impede your progress both when it arises and subsequently. In this case you would be unwise to affiliate too early with a lone medical director unless you are prepared to leave the area if you split—unless, of course, you are going to marry his daughter or he is guaranteed to retire or become disabled within one or two years. The second specific question you must answer is what type of hospital you wish to affiliate with. The hospital-based physician has a wide choice ranging from the small community hospital to the gigantic medical center. Stephen J. Miller, in *Prescription for Leadership*,[37] makes a strong case that the more prestigious the institution the more limited is the route to the top. In discussing the "medical elite," Miller demonstrates that, to become a department head in a university center, it is imperative to take your internship and residency in certain hallowed institutions of the eastern United States. So if that is your long-term goal, read Miller's book as early in your career as possible in order to make the necessary course corrections.

The entire subject of attaining the chairmanship of a major department in university medical centers or affiliated teaching hospitals is a fascinating study in practical politics. The career affiliations you make during your training are of paramount importance in including you in or excluding you from consideration for such eminence in the later stages of your career. The passing of the torch from one institution to another as a source of future department chairmen is based largely upon the determination of the current chief to help his boys get to the top. There are eminent subspecialists who are excellent teachers and whose only concern is to teach, and there are a lesser number who are equally concerned with the products of their teaching and so are highly selective in the affiliations they allow and the career plans of those they assist.

Although that has little to do with the usual hospital-based physician, the information you gain by talking to your peers in other fields may underscore the importance of some of these human relation factors that you might otherwise have ignored. Additionally, your peers may give you the clues to recognize a man in your own area of specialty who would be apt to treat and train you as his protégé. If you are unaware of this opportunity and pass it by, what you have lost may be of great concern to you in subsequent years. Maintain contact with all of the influential people in medicine with whom you have interacted significantly, and not merely those in your own narrow field of interest. Their viewpoints on events and possible help at critical moments may be invaluable to you in your efforts to cipher out what exactly is going on.

Returning to the medical specialties, if you are willing to pass up the chairmanship of a major department, you probably have a far wider range of options. Positions for which competition is less intense are theoretically available in wide array. They include the county hospitals, the Veterans Administration hospitals, and a number of other tax- and foundation-supported institutions. As you can quickly ascertain by reading the classified ads in the medical journals, geographical locations and institutional affiliations are prime determinants of just how desirable these positions are. Hospitals in desirable urban centers will have as keen competition for the department chairman's position as the universities; those in small isolated communities will have far less. In fact, positions in tax-supported institutions in small communities where remuneration is fixed but workload is not are generally available to anyone with the expertise and training.

If your plan is to become medical director of a department, you could do far worse than take a subsidiary position at a county or VA hospital with or without a preliminary period at the staff level. Your experience as you move up into the department head position will enhance your desirability when you come to compete for a position in a larger community hospital. If you have indeed made good use of the experience, you will be far better suited for managing departments at other hospitals. Additionally, it may be an ideal base for entrance into the mainstream of medical practice in the community, because you are entering from a strictly neutral position. That, however, assumes there is no major political infighting going on at the institution.

If you aim for the directorship in your specialty in a community hospital for reason of the additional open-ended financial advantages, you can proceed either directly or via one of the above alternatives. The danger in trying for a position in a hospital immediately upon leaving a training program is that your experience may be far too limited to enable you to do an effective job in the area of human relations. Achieving the position you desire too soon may actually derail your career if you fail to achieve the goals you publicly set. You may fool yourself that you are in an exalted position because of your abilities, whereas in fact you are there only because no one was available to challenge you. Thus when—inevitably—the challenger does come, you may be totally unprepared and react in a personal and self-defeating fashion.

Yet you are damned if you do and damned if you don't. This type of chance may come, you are told, only once in your lifetime; and if you do not seize it now, you may never have that opportunity again. An even worse dilemma, in the fields in which demand far exceeds supply, is to be presented such an opportunity before the essential portions of training are completed. Acceptance now may later lead to career jeopardy as more qualified physicians become available in that area.

THE OPENING MOVE

Let us assume that you are presently occupying an assistant's position in the area in which you would like to settle and that your performance is reasonably satisfactory. Either through your chief or, more likely, through the county medical association you may be assigned to the "speakers bureau"—one of the various specialty and county medical association activities that provide speakers for hospital educational programs. You are more likely to receive such an assignment if you are in a highly specialized field and if you are doing some original research work with your chief or on your own. Additionally, you must volunteer; no one is going to seek you out.

In any event, you should leap at every opportunity to speak for one very good reason: to display your wares. While you may be relying on your chief's contacts to line up something for you in the future, there is an advantage to developing a constituency of your

own. Even if the meeting is not in an area that interests you, remember the tremendous intricacies of human relations in all
societies. One of them is that physicians in private practice are
characteristically on the staffs of more than one hospital. In addition, physicians tend to associate with other physicians of similar
interests; and if someone is particularly impressed by your performance, he may drop the right word into the right ear at the
right time.

When you are asked to address a diverse group of physicians on
a specialty topic, you have in essence already been identified as the
expert. Thus there is no need to give a talk that is brilliant but
incomprehensible to your audience. If you want to be a department
head in a community hospital, one of the attributes you must exhibit is the ability to communicate clearly to your peers. If you talk
down to a group of gentlemen, you may not induce any recruitment fever. That is a terribly important point because many physicians, no doubt thanks to their own sense of inferiority or uncertainty, tend to overdo their talks to prove how much they know.
Instead of working out a fourth-order differential equation on the
blackboard for your awed audience, you should get across three or
four major and clinically useful points. Those points should be
eminently practical and applicable in their own local circumstances
by your audience. If after hearing you the members of that audience do not go back and do a better job, you have accomplished
very little.

If you proceed along the speaker's route, at some time someone
who hears you will be privy to the fact that a position requiring
your talent is about to come open. Positions in the non-tax-
supported institutions are rarely advertised because they are usually filled quickly by local or regional talent. There are enough
well-trained physicians in most specialty fields in the United States
today that no one need look too far to find a potentially competent
medical director. Only through audiences such as described here
can you increase the likelihood of having your name brought up for
consideration of some new position.

Obviously such a combination educational and public relations event is not fortuitous, but planned, and it requires continued efforts to implement it. You attended a meeting and addressed the audience in a manner that impressed and informed them and also subtly made known that you might be available if something interesting came up. (Obviously, you do not openly broach the subject in your talk, but in the subsequent one-to-one discussions it is not at all difficult to let people know about your possible availability.) The person who has the decision-making power may hear you directly or hear of you indirectly, and the game is now ready to proceed to stage two.

Beware of the perils of one-up-manship. When you speak in public forum, never answer even the stupidest question insultingly. No matter how delightful the retort that springs to your lips, restrain yourself; your purpose there is not to win a prize for debating. You may not have succeeded in putting the point across, so the question may not in fact be stupid at all. Even if the question is unnecessary, the questioner may be a potential contact or an influential person at a hospital in which you might be interested. If a heckler in the audience annoys you with one stupid question after another, ask him to come to see you after the meeting so you can help clear up his confusion without holding up the rest of the audience. There may be some interested spectators who are assessing your ability to perform under fire and to work with difficult members of the medical staff.

The personal satisfaction from a put-down is immediate, but the long-term costs are unknown. If you cannot foresee them, you had best forgo your smart retort. It is also useful to know just who is that person who is asking those questions; for his identity may tell you how to handle the problem. In this context I would recommend Dr. J. Ludwig's "A Letter to the Next Speaker."[38] Dr. Ludwig very aptly summarizes the major faults of inexperienced speakers and makes a number of useful and practical suggestions.

Unless you are an exceptionally vain person in a very rare specialty, there are likely to be present at these meetings members of your fraternity whom you should try to contact. In advance of your appearance it is wise to find out as much as you can about who is to be present. During your discourse you may even mention specific members of the audience as persons who are doing work in your area of interest. Such courtesies nearly always return dividends that you cannot anticipate; for in extending them you identify yourself as an ally rather than a rival. The persons you mention may even be the ones who have invited you to speak. Indeed, they may be the instigators of a search for a department chief, since they clearly recognize they cannot fulfill the task required by that position.

If you are in a specialty so unique that there is not yet a society for it, you can still find out who is working in that field. You can ask your former chief to begin with; beyond that you can call the various hospitals in your area and ask to speak to the technician in charge of that service or department. He can tell you who is doing the work. You can also call the medical staff office of various hospitals and ask them to give you the names of the people who are certified or claim expertise in your area of interest. If you take the time and the trouble to find out, you may discover the number of people acquainted with your field of interest is larger than you would have imagined. Now, these people can either be your potential boosters or your potential rivals. Your initial move determines which they will be.

As physicians, when confronted by a complex problem, we are trained to develop all of the pertinent information before we make an irrevocable decision, and it is repeatedly surprising to me that we so often ignore that training in the way we conduct our professional careers. The following is a case in point. A subspecialist takes a position in a tax-supported institution and, after one or two years, decides that he would like to go out into the community. Until that time, he has made no effort to contact anyone in the community apart from a few personal friends. He obtains from the Yellow Pages or the Hospital Council a list of hospitals in the area and their addresses. Next he composes a form letter detailing his interest in establishing or taking over Department X, encloses curriculum vitae, and fires his mailing off to the administrators of all the hospitals. He then sits back and waits for the offers to roll in.

Although that may not be a bad idea if the area is devoid of talent in his field, it is an unwitting insult if anyone qualified in that specialty is already present. The usual response of the hospital administrator upon receipt of such a letter is to turn it over to the incumbent medical director. Thus in one blow the prospective director has alienated a physician who might otherwise have been a useful ally and warned him that someone might be out after his position. Some hospitals have medical directors whom the administrators would like to replace, but it is highly unlikely that a shotgun letter will arrive on the very day that the administrator decides to act.

If you must proceed without advice from your chief—who may not know the area himself—and if you are not certain of your ground, the wisest approach is to call all the local physicians who are working in your field of interest. Speak frankly and tell them that you are presently occupying a position that you anticipate will be temporary and that you are looking for a more permanent post in their area. It may be that the physician to whom you are speaking needs help or knows of someone else who needs help or knows of an opportunity that he cannot himself pick up and that presents no threat to him. If you can thus ally yourself with another man in the field rather than identify yourself as a competitor, your subsequent career may be far more propitious than it otherwise might be.

THE FIRST CONTACT

Once you have made your availability known, hopefully to someone in a position of authority who acknowledges an opening, you will obviously wish to discuss the possibilities in some further detail. At this point, however, you must be careful that you are dealing not merely with a busybody, but with someone who has the authority to negotiate. In almost all hospitals that is the administrator; it is he who, with or without the chief of staff's consent, awards the contract. Therefore, be wary of discussing details of the position with anyone except the administrator or an accredited deputy. Your first response to an inquiry should be a request for some form of communication from either the administrator of the hospital or the current chief of staff with details of the position. You may find that the position is not actually open to you. Competing for a closed position will do nothing but generate ill will that may later bear bitter fruit. If you do not hear from the administrator either directly or indirectly, you should seriously question the validity of the offer; and do not respond with anything written to something less than a formal offer.

Once a formal offer has been made, you must obviously have a face-to-face meeting with the principals. Preliminary to that, however, must be your dispatch of certain documents. Your curriculum vitae and bibliography are not enough. If you are to be seriously in the running for the post of medical director, you should also include an outline of what you can do for the hospital as its director of Department X. The outline should include the various options that the hospital may choose from the services that you have available, as well as observations about the future course of development in that field.

The outline is a most important document, since it will demonstrate that you have a clear, concise, and organized mind and are in fact oriented toward management and leadership. Although such a statement may not impress the medical staff as much as the details of your specialty training would, it certainly will impress the administrators, most of whom have grave doubts about the ability of physicians to handle hospital staff and departments with any facility. Your curriculum vitae should elaborate upon any experience you have had in the management of groups. That may merely be a task force directed toward a particular problem, a project with some membership, or the assistantship of a department with a direct management activity. In any case, elaborate upon it; for it is the kind of

role for which you are applying and you must show that you have
had some appropriate experience.

BLIND ALLEYS

The Directorship positions in the clinical medical
specialties probably afford more opportunity for abuse than those
of the traditional departments. A common form of abuse that the
prospective director should learn to recognize and avoid is reduction to either the puppet or the unofficial house officer. Ideally the
medical director of a department acts as consultant, chief of the
service, and chairman of the appropriate committee. So if in discussing details of an opening the candidate finds out that (1) the
total clinical activity of the area in question is in the hands of a
group of practicing specialists, (2) they, not he, will answer all the
consultation requests, (3) one of them is titular head of the service,
(4) one of them is chairman of the committee, (5) the director will
have no direct powers of decision with regard to personnel, equipment, and budget, yet (6) he is supposed to take a badly organized,
staffed, and functioning department and radically improve it, he
should have qualms. If he wishes to dig further, the director-to-be
will learn that members of this group have been too preoccupied
with clinical activity to superintend or manage the department. What
he is involved in, beneath the surface, is an agreement between the
group and the administration to use up the skills of an anticipated
series of physician directors to upgrade the department while they
are being screened for suitability. Eventually, the most suitable
might be asked to join the group when they need another man.

The hazard of being "used up" is in marked contrast to the
underutilized position of director (puppet). Here the problem is not
too little to do, but too much, particularly after prime-time hours.
The director will find that he has too many consultations. A large
number will be for trivial reasons plus "And by the way, could
you . . .?" The requests will be for such services as monitoring,
starting IV's, following patients on the weekend, and answering

emergency calls. Once he finds other physicians signing out to him without his acquiescence ("Have Dr. B see Patient C for . . . and follow"), he will realize that what the medical staff wanted, and got, at very little expense, is a super house officer who, since he is billing for some of the services, cannot complain or demand reasonable hours. In both instances the base line remuneration from the hospital will be at the lower end of the scale.

YOUR IMAGE

The negotiations will be with the power group of the hospital, characteristically an older and more conservative group. These older, dynamic, aggressive men are used to having things their way. They do not tolerate differences, often including differences of a minor degree. How you appear in dress and manner to them is of prime importance. Although as a trainee or assistant in a tax-supported institution you might have had total freedom of dress and manner, the situation now facing you is different. The decision to award or not to award the post of medical director can hinge as easily upon the length of your hair or the number of expletives in your speech as upon your training, experience, and references. Your mode of dress may have nothing to do with your professional capability and competence, but your chances of demonstrating those capabilities professionally may depend very much on it, particularly during the first few meetings and encounters. Medicine is a hygienic profession, so you obviously should not appear unwashed or unkempt. The same stricture applies to your language. Older physicians are very straight; and though you may be perfect in everything else, your current mode of language use may be the factor that turns the tide.

After attending to your appearance, the next most important step in the first meetings is to listen with keen attention to everything that is said by those with whom you are meeting. Let them set the tone of the discussion and let them do the talking. In general, the one who talks the most reveals the most. By keeping your comments to a minimum, you retain more freedom of action. You have already sent in your curriculum vitae and your outline of proposed services; there is little more that you need to discuss about yourself personally. What you need now is to learn all you can about the people who are considering you for a post.

THE POSITION OFFERED

Once you are certain that the position offered is real, the next question is whether you want it on the terms presented. At this point, the issue is less financial than it is a matter of the politics and philosophy of the power group offering the position. After adequate discussion, you must ask yourself whether you can work with these men comfortably for the next ten years. If your experience tells you that the answer is no, you had better graciously decline so as not to waste both your time and theirs. Your decisiveness in rejecting an unsuitable position may impress someone who has something better to offer in the future. Certainly, if you decline, you must give an acceptable reason as a basis for your decision to forestall any hostility.

If, on the other hand, you decide you can work with these men, negotiations can begin in earnest. Your negotiating approach will vary with the circumstances. If you are brought in secretly to discuss a position still occupied by someone else, then you really are in a disadvantageous position. No matter how good the offer sounds on paper, you must be able to circulate about the hospital, meet the people with whom you would be interacting, talk about the department, and gain information that will enable you to plan accordingly. In addition, by acceding to the request for *sub rosa* negotiations and agreement you set a precedent that will make it very difficult for you later to change the mode of your negotiations with the hospital and the medical staff. And what they did to your predecessor they can do as easily to you.

Hopefully the agreement and the search will be aboveboard. If there is an incumbent, he knows he is on his way out and is available to meet you. It is highly advisable politically to talk with him to find out what the story is from his point of view. Also, you must inspect the hospital in detail and depth including your own particular department and all the departments with which your department will most closely interact. If you are clinically oriented, you should visit all of the clinical facilities and speak to their key personnel. After a preliminary tour in the company of the administrator, it is wise to return on your own later and speak informally with the various key middle-management people. Preferably that will be in a casual setting over coffee to get a better idea of what is going on in that department and in the rest of the hospital.

THE PREAGREEMENT SURVEY

Logic, and not paranoia, is the reason for a complete survey of the department before you accept any position. If you are obligated, in your agreement with the hospital, to perform certain tasks, you must be assured that the necessary resources are present and operational. That means you must survey the department for its weak and strong points, especially in the area of personnel. It is worthwhile to set forth on paper the deficiencies that you have identified and that must be corrected immediately if you are to conduct the department affairs to the satisfaction of yourself and the hospital.

Your cognizance of all these departmental minutiae cannot be left until the negotiations are completed and a document is signed. Hospital administrators are under tremendous pressure from all sides to meet escalating needs; they can meet only a portion of all the necessary demands. Verbal promises to do something about the deficiencies in your department will have little validity if some greater, more urgent need arises. If there are substandard elements in the department, they must be corrected. Have it written into your agreement. Otherwise, you will be hounded and bounded by the substandard items for as long as administration dodges the issue.

Almost certainly you will be asked to speak to the medical staff for a variety of reasons: (1) for you to meet them and for them to see you in action, (2) for them to listen to you, see what you know, see how you come on, (3) for them to see how you handle yourself in the stress of a new situation, and (4) most importantly, for you to determine what it is they expect you to do for them. As mentioned above, you should discuss practical matters with the staff, since the presumed reason for your arrival is to conduct the department in as efficient a manner as is practicable. You can mention that there are many more esoteric matters you could discuss and promise a lecture series on them for those who are interested, but limit your current topics to specifics of what you will do, what you can do, and what you will not be able to do.

Even if on your initial visits everything seems tremendously appropriate and you can foresee no problem, you should not formally accept the position until you have had some time to consider it and to discuss it with your spouse, family, and legal adviser. Use the interval to confirm all the good things you've heard about the place, as well as to check out the degree of understatement regarding the less attractive things you have heard. You also need to discuss the long-term implications of the decision with your spouse and hopefully arrive at a common viewpoint.

YOUR IMPLIED CONTRACT WITH THE MEDICAL STAFF

Your assumption of the post of director implicitly obligates you to perform in the interest of the medical staff of that hospital. The only possible exception is in the tax-supported institution, where the organizational structure is such that the medical staff is essentially powerless. In that one instance, you may operate independently of the wishes of the medical staff, but only at your own risk. The political realities are such that in all cases you should look for a mandate from the medical staff in the performance of your duties.

The secret to a long-term stable relationship is to provide the staff with all the germane services that they require. This means you must find out from them the services they need rather than egotistically assume that, because you are the expert, you know full well what everyone should want. That egotistical assumption is one of the major pitfalls that many directors stumble into because their training has in no way made them consumer-oriented—even when the consumers are other physicians.

Thus the medical director urgently needs feedback from all members of the medical staff who utilize the department to confirm that the product is indeed what the prescribers wished and that desired areas of service are not left untouched. In fact, if you are putting allocated funds into expansion, you must be certain that the expansion is in areas needed by the staff, not those in which you have a purely personal interest. The consequence of spending considerable sums of money for the benefit of neither the hospital nor the medical staff is less money next time you ask.

Your preliminary survey during the negotiating period, if conducted properly and in adequate depth, will give you a reasonably good idea of what is presently needed to correct significant deficiencies. On the basis of your training and experience, you can then enlarge on what else might be done. Those conclusions, of course, should be amalgamated into your original report. The report should not merely sit on the administrator's desk or in his file; it should circulate among the decision-making councils of the medical staff. You need to have, on paper, an outline of the things done and the things you propose to do so that you can find out from the doctors whether that is really what they want and whether anything is missing. Of course, there will be a number of pie-in-the-sky services that they would like to see. Your continuing dialogue with them should gradually evolve a priority system for services—actual, projected, and pie-in-the-sky—in the coordinated long-range development plan and budget projection.

One of the prime means of gaining insight into departmental needs is to obtain a list of the top ten or fifteen users of your department's services. Although the ten or fifteen will be only a small percentage of the total number of doctors using your department, it will undoubtedly represent a major fraction of services consumed. It is a group with whom you have a reasonably good chance of meeting and discussing, on an individual basis, the future of the department's services. As the heaviest consumers of your product, their input should be incorporated into your immediate and long-range plans and then taken back to the entire staff for validation and approval.

THE IMPACT OF PRECEDENT

A disastrous habit common to young medical directors is a failure to recognize the impact of precedent. When a new man enters, all the onlookers closely watch his reaction to day-to-day occurrences. Trouble arises when the director reacts variably to certain situations, with the result that consternation and confusion ensue among the participants and onlookers. That does not mean the director must develop a frozen standard operating procedure for every conceivable situation. It merely means that he should give careful attention to his response to each situation that he meets for the first time in order to evolve a response that he can comfortably repeat subsequently. He certainly can alter his pattern of response if the situation changes, but he must be sure that the situation, and not merely his perception of it, really is different and get that point across to his audience.

Precedent establishes credibility because the other participants can rely upon certain events following in sequence. Once you begin to destroy precedent, you erode your credibility as well. Each situation deserves not only a careful analysis of its present components but also a search of your memory for your response to the situation in the past.

One of the precedent-making activities is to set forth clearly, on paper, your proposed plans, activities, and analyses of situations. The very adoption of the language of management sets an important precedent, since you are dealing not only with the medical staff of the hospital but also with its management. Another important precedent involves your relations with your peers, particularly if you are board-certified and they are not. In this day of rules and regulations, that slip of paper is important to those without official notice of status as specialists; it puts them very much on the defensive and thus more likely to react emotionally under stress.

Of course, the worth of a man cannot be encompassed by a slip of paper, particularly in the field of medicine. There are board-certified physicians who are ossified, and there are board-eligible physicians who are still growing and learning. So you must establish the precedent of dealing with people on the level of their abilities rather than on the level of their credentials. The problem is more apt to arise if you are an associate to a medical director who is not board-certified whereas you are. But no matter how much you try to play it down, those without certification will always feel threatened by you and react appropriately. One of the skills you must demonstrate as manager is the ability to keep those prickly people working together rather than fighting and jockeying for advantage both within your department and throughout the hospital.

EXPANDING YOUR CONTRACT
WITH THE MEDICAL STAFF

The cornerstone of your contract with the medical staff is courtesy. That means listening before responding, replying rather than lecturing, and totally eschewing gamesmanship. If you act straight with the medical staff and are at all times helpful and essentially noncompetitive, then you not only strengthen your position with them but reinforce their need to deliver their part of the contract with you. The medical staff have a great tendency to ignore the reciprocal aspects of this implied contractual relationship, but your very consistency in delivery may press them into becoming as supportive of you as you are of them. That means specifically that they must keep you informed about the objective pluses and minuses in your department's performance and that they must cooperate with you when you require their help in changing departmental performance.

Often it is the medical staff's long-time habits, rather than the departmental performance, that are the problem. Doctors frequently procrastinate and then complain about the technicians who attempt to pick up after them. Obviously, one way to overcome that failing is an effective educational program. Formal educational time with its large audiences, however, is limited. If you are frustrated by competing demands from other departments with equal priority for educational time, you must substitute another form of education, namely, the one-to-one teaching conference. That is a technique, "curbstone consult," that is widely used by older, more experienced men who seize upon almost every staff contact as an opportunity to both learn and teach. Merely by asking the doctor for information first, you may instruct him by changing his perspective of the problem. While not as prestigious, these methods of changing staff attitude are in most cases more effective than the formal lecture.

Another aspect of developing contracts with the hospital medical staff is your openness. Here precedent plays an important role. If you begin with secret deals, you are almost certain to be plagued with a continuing onslaught of them. There isn't a medical group around that won't be glad to get you into a corner and make a deal about a situation to their own advantage. Your only defense is to keep all negotiations as open as possible. Set the precedent of taking most grievances back to an open committee meeting. Then if you find yourself being squeezed or forced into an agreement that is really unconscionable, your defense is to have it out in the light of a committee discussion where everyone can look at it. Obviously, there are some technicalities—such as your exact remuneration, your relations with administration, and other technicalities concerning departmental management—that must be kept under wraps for political and personal reasons, but all else should be reasonably public information.

In this regard I would like to point out a simple precept that is ignored more often than it is observed: never say anything about anyone that would seriously embarrass you if it were repeated, particularly to the subject of your conversation. The number of human relations that have been soured by unnecessary sniping of someone else's perception of the problem is incalculable. You may be certain that, if you have a tendency to put down a person who is not there, your remarks will someday come home to roost.

Actually, to receive feedback on your performance from the

medical staff, you must develop increased insight into your own activities and the way you come on. It is so very easy to get people to tell you what you want to hear, because you are in a position to reward those who say the right things and punish those who say the wrong things. Most people cannot be bothered to get into a fight because they said something unpleasant; therefore, they will mouth pap or say nothing at all. When you are receiving no input at all from the medical staff or the input is in the category of pap, you had better wonder whether you are performing as well as you think.

The difficulty is to get someone to open up and tell you what the problems are. You may find, in the words of the famous slogan, that even your best friends won't tell you because they feel obligated to defend you. In so doing, however, they are actually sabotaging you. By not giving you feedback, they eliminate the chance that you will improve. Ultimately, most casual friendships erode under such continual underground dissatisfaction, and you suddenly find the majority turning on you.

7

REMUNERATION AND CONTRACTS

GENERAL PERSPECTIVE

A hospital-based physician is not in an ideal position to achieve maximum levels of income. Unless there are some very unusual circumstances, he will, after a lifetime of service at one or more hospitals, have little more to show for his career than his personal estate, the money he has saved, and his memories. In contrast, the man who establishes an office to conduct primary care will have, in addition to the personal estate, money, and memories, the very real assets of a practice, accounts receivable, equipment, years of tax advantage, and possibly investment in a building. Thus the hospital-based physician must be willing to trade off loss of income potential for some other benefits, and security is not one of them. The physician in practice is the one who is more secure; for it is difficult, provided he remains marginally competent, to remove him from his financial base of support once he is well established.

The advantages of a medical directorship include such nonpecuniary factors as the freedom to pursue other activities, a free hand in developing services one is interested in, investigational activities, publishing activities and teaching opportunities, and the freedom to change one's interests radically in response to new needs in the environment. Those opportunities are not readily accessible to the physician in private practice, since his first and greatest priority is the care of his patients.

There are some questions the embryo specialist should ask before he actually embarks on such a career pattern. First, is the field well established with a great deal of talented competition? If so, you had better be resigned to a long career as someone else's assistant. Although you may receive substantial monetary reward, you may also have to coexist as a high-class indentured servant of a domineering older physician. The only alternative is to move into areas that are far less attractive but in which there are openings.

Second, if you are going into a relatively new field, are you flexible enough to adjust and to withstand the additional strains of developing in an area with few guidelines? Finally, if yours is a field with a clinical orientation, rather than a purely diagnostic one, what do you expect to be doing in ten and twenty years—clinical work or purely departmental work? You may have to make such a choice or else have it made for you. True, you may choose the paperwork route to eminent status, salary, and prestige, but in five or ten years your clinical skills will be sadly depleted should you wish to switch back into the alternative career pattern of active practice of medicine. Although quite obviously no one can predict exactly what he will want to be doing in five or ten years, the choices you make now will inevitably influence the options available to you later.

AVAILABLE INCOME SOURCES

There are a variety of ways in which a physician can be compensated for his services, but the type of compensation depends on the type of service provided and the opportunities present. As an associate, your compensation will probably be limited to a straight salary. In subsequent years you may be able to enlarge the manner in which you generate income, depending upon your relationship with the man who employs you. If you are in a field with a plentiful supply of young recently trained competitors, you almost certainly will run into senior men who will gladly employ you for a limited salary for short periods of time. Contrary to expectations, once you have demonstrated your worth by the excellence of your work and your value to the department, you may find yourself dumped rather than having your one-year contract renewed. That is due not to a personal grudge but to just simple good business. The senior man finds it advisable to change his associates before they become too expensive and are potential competitors.

That pattern is possible only in areas in which medical skills can be provided without much physician-to-physician contact and is more apt to be found in such diagnostic fields as radiology and pathology. There you will have to possess far more than mere finely honed technical skills if you are to achieve any of your goals, one of which I would presume to be stability. One way to achieve stability is to enlarge your experience in your early career; you rapidly move through a series of positions to age and mature yourself in an accelerated fashion. If you are near the right spot at the right time, someone may remember you and call you if you have been effective.

Of course, if you move in and out too rapidly, the medical staff may never get to know you well enough to remember you when need arises. But even here it is your nontechnical abilities, namely, human relations and public relations, that will determine whether you receive the call.

Departmental directors potentially have available to them a far greater variety of methods of remuneration than their assistants. The choices open will depend upon your geographical locations, the circumstances in your particular specialty, and the previous history of that institution and of its sister institutions in that area. Some of these options are:

1. Salaried position in a community hospital, either part- or full-time.
2. Independent contractor in a community hospital.

3. Associate/partner/owner of a service company that provides your specialty's services to that hospital.
4. A salaried or retainer position with a group of physicians, but assigned to act as director of a hospital department to the mutual benefit of that group or clinic and the institution.
5. A civil service employee position.
6. "Voluntary" medical director with the proviso that you will derive your income from consultations and the further implication that all possible consultations will be sent to you.
7. Voluntary medical director with an outside income source either grant or other institutional support.

Only the second and third options (namely, independent contractor or associate/partner/owner of a service company) offer you the possibility of earning a potentially very large income. The sixth option, voluntary medical director living on clinical work, is really a very poor choice, since it forces one to rely upon income-producing activities to the detriment of departmental interests. Thus at some point in time it is likely that the medical staff will seek someone who can do the management job properly.

YOUR STATUS AS AN INDEPENDENT CONTRACTOR

An independent contractor status entails an agreement with a hospital to share the risk with regard to your income. As your income is geared to departmental activity, you can have no assurance as to its exact amount. The agreement obligates you to provide specified services in return for a share of the departmental income. The key words are "obligation to provide services," and in contrast to salaried positions, contractual obligations such as this have no time limits. The obligation, unless specifically limited in the contract, could apply 24 hours a day, 365¼ days a year. In addition, no matter how low the income falls, you remain under contract to provide the service until readjustment or agreement termination. Before you undertake such an obligation, you had best be certain that it is something that you can fulfill either directly or with help.

You can avoid that open-ended obligation by choosing a lower level of independent contractor status, namely, that of technical adviser to the department. As technical adviser, you receive a retainer, not a salary. The hospital pays you as a specialist in your professional sphere for advice and services or in return for a claim upon your services in case of need. Since your only obligation is to be available for those services, you can do something else with the free time, provided you can drop the other activity when contractual need arises.

Those who wish to receive income proportionate to their output usually do so by arranging to receive a percentage of departmental net or gross income. In recent years, many state boards of medical examiners have assumed a conflict-of-interest situation when a doctor has requested a percentage of the net, since he might be tempted to reduce the quality of care to improve his share. Thus the common arrangement is a percentage of the gross. The physician who dislikes so direct a relation between productivity and income can choose more indirect approaches, such as a percentage based on the number of days he is at the hospital, the various items of the department's product, or even the number of hours he puts in at the job.

The hours-on-the-job alternative has little to recommend it. Undoubtedly you will put in far more hours than you had originally anticipated; and unless you carry a timecard, it will be hard to justify or prove the extra hours to the administrator. In addition, the administrator will look with great skepticism upon your request for payment for extra hours spent in the department's benefit outside the hospital. More often than not, your hours will be decided by the person who is paying on the basis of what he thinks you are doing. Also, if you tie your income to anything other than the dollars earned by the department, you effectively eliminate any cost-of-living increases. In general, if it is the dollars you are interested in, it is best to have your income tied in with the dollars that the department generates.

A common mistake made by physicians who choose the independent contractual approach is to assume that the income from the hospital contract is actually their personal gross salary. In years to come, as departmental income increases, your contract will award you more money, but you may be doing the same or even less work for it. If at the start you receive $x for y hours of service, then when the contract income goes up to $3x you may have trouble explaining why you are still providing only y hours, unless you were grossly underpaid at the outset. The obligation laid upon an independent contractor is that he will provide additional help services as growing utilization generates additional rewards. That means either you yourself will provide more hours of work (or items of service) or you will get additional help to provide new services so that the increased income will be offset by increased services to the hospital.

The major benefit from this type of arrangement is that it automatically provides the funds for additional help when the department has grown. Since those funds are controlled by you, rather than by someone else, you can divert them as quickly as you wish to additional help without fighting about budget or time allocation. The difficulty is to retain your objectivity about departmental needs that you should be satisfying. It is very tempting to say that as you age you are worth more and therefore you should keep more; but there may be people in power who disagree with that, particularly if your imagined improved services are just that, imagined. You must provide irrefutable objective evidence of increased services as increased income is generated. That principle should have the status of an absolute law with each independent contractor.

CONFLICT OF INTEREST

Serious conflict of interest may arise at a number of levels in the hospital. Most important to the medical director are those involving medical staff interests. Conflict is more apt to arise in areas in which clinical services are part of the departmental product. There sometimes is a thin line between doing the hospital's work and doing your own work on the hospital's time. What is more, that line may vary from season to season, depending on the needs of the community.

In some cases, it is actually negligent not to provide clinical services on what could otherwise be classified as hospital time, owing to the tremendous demand and need for such services by the staff. In such cases, of course, one must make appropriate adjustments by providing an equivalent value of service to compensate for any advantage gained by the clinical activity. If the director has the time and energy to provide services only where demand is greatest, he will eventually end up in a gross violation of his agreement because that greatest demand is always in the area of patient care. Hospital departments normally operate from 9:00 to 5:00, Monday through Friday, although in clinical services the coverage may extend throughout the entire 24 hours of each day, 7 days a week.

However, most contracts with physicians assume the so-called prime-time coverage. Thus, if the hospital is indeed remunerating you adequately for your prime-time activities on their behalf, both administration and the medical staff will quickly recognize unfair advantage taken when you use that time on income-producing activities for your personal benefit. If you have a patient in the hospital whom you must follow, it may be necessary to see him during prime time, but hopefully you will find a way to replace those minutes taken from hospital time.

A related violation is the use of the department to solicit or obtain private patients for the director, either direct care or consultation cases. That is more apt to be a problem when there are physicians in your specialty who are available but who, because of their lack of connection with the department, have less demand for their services than you do as director. Equally bad over the long term is the problem of specific patient care. If both you and another physician in your specialty are taking care of patients with the same problems but your patients receive better in-hospital care and attention because your department responds that way, the differential will be noted and more than commented upon.

In both instances, you must avoid a posture in which it is obvious that you have unfair advantage. The other physicians are earning money only when they are providing patient care. If you are earning the same patient income as they are, as well as hospital income, you may be sure that someday that will be discussed in a manner that is not going to be useful to your long-term plans.

OPTIONS

The salaried position, although limited in income prospects, has many advantages that the independent contractor status has not. It is more beneficial to the specialists who know in advance that they will have difficulty finding additional help. Since your health is always essential to long-term activity, restricting your obligations from the start may be a wise choice. In general, your obligations in terms of hours are far fewer, since as department head the extra hours are related more to unusual than to regular demand. Thus you are entitled to weekends, holidays, sick time, educational and vacation activities, and leave of absence without jeopardizing your position.

Whether the hospital is able to provide coverage during those absences is as much their problem as yours; certainly for a fixed salary you need not provide the same coverage that an independent contractor must. However, as a salaried physician in a community hospital, you are on an even more conspicuous spot when it comes to conflict of interest with regard to fee-for-service patient care. Here especially you must avoid the implication that you are using your salaried hours to take care of private pay patients.

When the demand for services is especially keen owing to the shortage of trained specialists, there may be additional opportunities for deals. If an institution, usually a tax-supported county hospital, has an opening at a lower salary than is commonly earned by doctors at that specialty level, someone in authority often "compromises" by hiring a specialist and paying him for eight hours while requiring that he provide only six or fewer hours of service. Although that procedure has long-term disadvantages to the institution, it may or may not be disadvantageous to the physician. Certainly he can use the position to keep his skills available in that area while he uses the extra time to find a more desirable position locally.

The danger here is the temptation to reduce your hours to five, four, three, two, or one. The consequences of such negligence will be determined by the degree of abuse and by the extent of administrative surveillance of the physician's activities. Now in the short term that may be tolerated if the original incumbent uses the time he has "misappropriated" to make an opening for himself in the community and recruit, as soon as he can, an assistant or associate to fill the civil service position and provide the hours contractually agreed upon. The community ultimately is benefited if there are now two specialists where before there were none.

The advantage of a salaried position is that it limits your time commitment. In fact, you may use the budgeted time to try to develop a position for an assistant or associate. Obtaining help in that way invariably takes far longer than through the independent contractor approach. However, it does offer a buffer between you and the tide of increased demand that you do not feel capable of meeting solely by your own efforts. The difficulty is that if the need for your services increases dramatically, you may have to become bureaucratic in your restrictions on what it is you will do—and you may or may not be in a strong enough position to make those restrictions hold. The added workload always arrives before help does, so you may be assured of a state of continuing dilemma for some time.

Another problem with a department in which each physician is salaried is that the director may not have the necessary control; for once his associate has tenure, he can operate independently rather than as a member of a team and thereby aggravate rather than help the director. If in the independent contractor situation the assistant does not work out, the contractor can, much more expeditiously, remove him from the scene and search for a more suitable replacement. The problem of altered behavior of an employee who has attained tenure is an ongoing civil service dilemma. Obviously, the selection process for a position in which tenure is a factor must be even more searchingly thorough than that in which a dissident can be removed at any time.

THE SERVICE COMPANY

At a certain stage in the development of new departments, forming a service company may be a logical step. When a new area of service is beginning to bud, there really is no market for a full-time specialist; even with clinical work, he will have time on his hands. When that point has been reached, an entrepreneur may contract with a group of hospitals to provide the new service. He will then recruit the necessary technical and medical personnel. The arrangement is more apt to occur in newer clinically oriented services such as gastroenterology, pulmonary diseases, and renal dialysis.

Servicing the needs of several institutions will provide sufficient demand to support a pool of talent as well as the necessary equipment. But the physician who handles the medical aspects of the service should be aware that, unless he has a piece of the action, he is merely another talent to be used to the company's advantage. Now if the director himself has set up the company, he controls the financial as well as the medical activity and so is in a far more advantageous position. In fact, there are cases in which the director has established and then sold the service company, including his talents, to a larger more economically based organization, in return for salary and stock options. But unless you share the profits of such a company, recognize that, since the company exists to make money, it will use you.

A further disadvantage is that, if your services are split up among a large number of institutions, you may find that the quality of the product you provide is eroded by the time you spend in transit. That may damage your reputation far more than that of the company and may actually reduce your attractiveness to the medical community.

THE VOLUNTARY STATUS OPTION

Voluntary status is a treacherous option. Success depends upon the medical director's ability to quickly establish lasting, binding relations and alliances with the medical staff and administration. Moreover, if he is successful, he will usually work himself out of a job; for as he generates the clinical activity to give him the income he needs, he will find he has less and less time for the department. The consequence may be that he creates a position for some other physician who comes in as either an ally or a competitor. Particularly if the director is not able to enlist or develop a well-trained, middle-level management supervisor, he may find that his reputation as department director will suffer. Also, the pressure always remains that, if he is unable to maintain his professional relations with the majority of the medical staff, his source of consultative patient material may dry up when newer, more attractive talent enters the area.

The only circumstance in which the voluntary status option might be useful is when an area has two or more hospitals in keen competition for patients. Hospital A subsidizes a director in establishing a practice and a department to attract the local medical staff. The director may one day negotiate with Hospital B about starting a department there, with an excellent financial arrangement, because he can bring along the large patient population that he acquired at Hospital A.

Of course, that is a polite form of coercion, but it does work when approached on a pragmatic, long-term basis. The director is in a position of power, since there is always one hospital that needs the patients that only he can supply. The difficulty arises when the director becomes so busy clinically that he cannot perform the departmental functions required of him. Then the department grows, not in breadth of services, but merely in expansion of the present level of utilization for the director's own patients. Ultimately, to satisfy the medical staff, the director will need to get an associate to run the department. If the associate is sufficiently energetic and astute, he may, once he is established in the community, move over to the competing hospital and set up an adequate department that will draw other physicians back.

A variation of the voluntary option is for the physician to join a clinic group that has an arrangement with a hospital. The physician makes his financial arrangements with the clinic, and his duties include responsibility for the hospital department. More often than not, any rewards for his activities will be paid to the clinic rather than to the director, so he in effect is building an empire for someone else.

Another problem is that his close association with the clinic group may wall him off from the rest of the medical community unless the clinic actually encompasses most of the hospital's medical staff. But if the clinic group is competing with a group of independent practitioners, it will be difficult for the director, unless he is especially skilled in human relations, to develop any form of following among or relations with the other physicians. That may nullify his efforts to develop the department no matter how bright the theoretical prospects for his work.

Physicians are perfectly capable of irrational behavior; they may refuse to use a service simply because they do not like the person in charge of it. Such a medical decision by even a small group of determined men generates economic pressures that may derail plans for the gradual development of a complete department. Particularly when the director is egotistical, immature, or dogmatic, the whole effort may be doomed to failure.

THE INCOME FLOOR

All variable methods of remuneration should explicitly include a minimum level of dollar support per month. Even if there is no activity in the department, a director must receive enough money to support himself and his essential professional activities. Otherwise, the director has no real obligation to perform during periods of extreme slowdown. Unless the hospital has first call on his services at all times, the director who is temporarily without significant income must inevitably shift his interest to a more profitable direction. Once that happens, the hospital is in danger of losing a man who could otherwise be a very considerable long-term asset. In several instances failure to recognize the need for an adequate minimal remuneration has led to loss of talent from an area with no readily available replacement.

GROWTH FACTORS IN THE AGREEMENT

Gentleman's agreements may be regarded as written in sand. Years later, under stress, there will be any number of recollections of what was agreed upon. The only predictable thing is a tremendous disagreement; for each party will feel certain of his own interpretation. That is most apt to happen with unwritten provisions for growth of coverage to meet growing demand for services. In the first place, the man you made the agreement with may or may not be there when the verbal clause must be invoked. His successor undoubtedly will have no memory of it, and he will be most unhelpful in taking your word for the agreement.

Only the independent contractor status automatically provides for the growth factor by supplying the additional income to satisfy it. All other arrangements require that you go back to the administration and try to crowbar loose additional funds for help. Depending upon the circumstances, you may or may not succeed. The problem is that, as income goes up, so does the hospital's utilization of it; and although the department's activity may have gone from x to $3x$, all the additional future income may have been allocated. Now, if you are in a position to receive a substantial fraction of that additional income yourself but do not regard all of it as rightfully yours, you can split off an appropriate portion of it to pay someone else. However, if you regard all of the growth income as your own, your right, and your due and must get still more from the hospital to pay that extra help, you may, of course, meet with a negative response.

You cannot afford to wait until you are swamped with work before you do something about looking for help. The problem of growth must be built into the initial agreement even though you can foresee no trend for growth at the time you insist upon arranging for it. Otherwise, you must devote time and effort to get the agreement modified at a time when you are already desperately pressed for any spare hours to fulfill your personal needs. And you must remember that, having obtained license to get the help, you must then devote additional time to searching out, recruiting, and breaking in.

CHOOSING YOUR LEGAL ADVISER

The medical professional is quite logical in his approach to his own field of expertise. No medical specialist would undertake a surgical procedure, and certainly no surgeon would electively undertake a procedure for which he had no specific training. Yet we characteristically find that physicians and surgeons attempt to do their own negotiating and make their own contractual arrangements as if they had been specifically trained to do so. If you have legal and business training, particularly in contract law, then you should do very well in negotiating for yourself. Otherwise, the advice of a mature, experienced, and appropriate expert can be invaluable in enabling you to see the long-term consequences of present decisions.

The money you save by getting free advice over the telephone from a friend of your in-laws is a pittance compared to the money you may lose if some astute administrator takes advantage of your naiveté. Just as a physician would call in the appropriate consultant on a problem that was clearly out of his field, so you should meet the same professional needs by calling in a consultant on a legal problem. Curbstone consults may be useful for a person with some awareness of what is involved; but certainly when no training or background is present, a full and formal approach is advisable.

The function of the consultant is not necessarily to do something new, but rather to provide a different viewpoint of the problem. What you most need is an independent perspective of your requirements, your needs, and the obligations of the position offered. Certainly you need to discuss all those matters with immediate family members in whom you normally confide, but you also need advice from someone who can be totally objective because he is not emotionally bound to you. You may be certain that the hospital administrator with whom you are negotiating has had either formal or practical contract negotiation training, and that, in addition, he will review all of the details of the agreement with his hospital's attorney.

Thus one of the first requirements of negotiation is to find a legal adviser who will be able to advise you appropriately. That is no easy matter if you are new in the area. Yet at that very stage the advice and help from a man who knows the area and its people can be of inestimable value. A well-placed attorney may be able to provide you with additional or supplementary information that will clarify puzzling aspects of your general talks with administration and medical staff. He may thus provide you, a newcomer in the area, with the experience you need to make long-range decisions. The less experienced and the less well acquainted you are with the area and its peculiarities, the more you need to rely upon his expertise. In fact, the neophyte medical director, to avoid serious missteps, will need to review with his attorney virtually all stages of development that require far-reaching decisions.

Even if you are merely to be an assistant or an associate, it is wise to have an attorney review the arrangement or contract. If the physician for whom you hope to work is unable to offer you anything specific, particularly in writing, you should offer to provide him with your written version of the agreement drawn up by your attorney to nail down the essential points. Regardless of how agreeable and gentlemanly the other party is, you must reduce the agreement to writing and have someone with the proper background examine it. Even a year's contract will involve $25,000 to $50,000 or more, far too large a sum to deal with casually.

The only time you may not need an attorney is when the position is that of a salaried or a civil service employee with fixed terms so that you can rely upon precedent and the experience of others to protect you from individual misfortune. Even then, however, there is room for individual bargaining, and you may by your lack of foresight miss some options that might have been available to you had you insisted upon discussing them. Even as a salaried employee you need to have some clear indication of your financial prospects in the future, particularly if your responsibilities and obligations are going to increase. If there is no recognition of the rising cost of living, the increased value of your services, or the fulfillment of additional obligations at the time you first enter into the agreement, you may be sure that you will have to fight for it in subsequent years.

Let us assume that you want to find an attorney but you do not know where to look. You have no contacts and you need a lawyer in a hurry because the administrator is pressing you to agree to certain things that puzzle and trouble you. You could call the local office of the Bar Association and be given the first name on the list for that day's referrals, but that is unlikely to find you the man most suited to your needs. You could go through the Yellow Pages and pick someone whose name impresses you. Both methods rely upon pure chance.

A more logical approach is to get suggestions from other medical directors at the hospital, call the attorneys, speak to them regarding your problems and your special circumstances, and ask who could be most suitable. In that way you will at least have the names of several attorneys who have done some medical staff contract work. All too often the neophyte says, "Well, since I am so inexperienced, let me get the very best there is." Here the practical problem is that the very best in the area may not be the best for you. He may be so busy that he cannot really give you the time and attention that your case requires. In all likelihood he will turn you over to an associate, if he has one, who may or may not be the very next best.

The attorney who is best for you will be one who, first of all, has been in practice for some time in the area so that he knows what is going on in the community. Second, he must be held in reasonably high repute by certain independent people such as bank managers, medical directors, accountants, and other attorneys.

Third, he must not be so busy that he does not have time for you, particularly to talk to you by telephone when urgent questions come up. Fourth, you need a man who will work with you and who is flexible.

The last stipulation is very important; for there are quite a number of attorneys who specialize in hospital contract work but whose major clients are pathologists and radiologists. That is fine if you are in one of those specialties. However, if you are in a much rarer specialty with unique problems of its own, you may find his approach counterproductive because he is operating by rote. Every time you try to explain your problems, he replies, "That's okay, I know all about it" when it is quite obvious he doesn't. It may be possible, however, to use such a man by asking him to help you find a younger attorney whom he knows personally and professionally and would recommend as someone who could develop in this line of experience. Hopefully the older man will have enough maturity to accept the fact that you are looking for someone else and assist you accordingly—just as a physician who isn't quite the right specialty may assist a patient in finding someone more appropriate to his needs.

CHECKING YOUR CHOICE

If you have the time, it is best to try out the man you have chosen on several small tasks such as the handling of a lease, a contract to purchase, or a will. Obviously, however, if you are already in the midst of a major contractual negotiation, you must proceed immediately to the problem at hand. But even at this point, you can assess his approach to the problem by determining whether he proceeds in as logical a fashion as you would in a problem in your field.

Begin by writing down all of the questionable points in the agreement that you are negotiating, including any unusual aspects of your relation to the hospital, and follow up with a series of questions about the items that are troubling you. If the attorney is then unable to obtain the additional information he needs, analyze the problem, and present you with logical answers and suggestions, you may have chosen the wrong man. He may have insufficient background information; he may be trying to solve a problem that is not your problem; he may not be communicating effectively; or he may simply be giving you too little attention. If you telephone him subsequently to obtain additional comments and he is always out and the only way to get an answer is to make another appointment, then he is probably not going to be useful to you at all. A man who is too busy to be reasonably available by telephone is probably going to be too busy to devote the time to your problem that is required.

The attorney needs to be directly involved with the other key people in the negotiation of a contract for several reasons. First, his presence at the time of negotiation gives the medical director an opportunity to evaluate how the attorney handles himself and the medical director's interests. Second, the attorney's assessment of the other people in the meeting may provide the medical director with useful insight. Third, just as a medical director evaluates the attorney's performance, so the attorney evaluates the medical director's role in a meeting and provides him with feedback and appropriate suggestions for conduct at subsequent meetings. Fourth, without his attorney the medical director will be effectively outnumbered even if he is negotiating one-to-one with the administrator, since the administrator's seniority and superiority of position give him a definite advantage. However, it is the medical director, not his attorney, who should conduct and set the tone of his part of the meeting. The attorney's role is not to lead the meeting or provoke a confrontation, but rather to provide backup and advice.

Once you have acquired sufficient experience, you can negotiate on a one-to-one basis with the administrator. Most administrators have negotiated so many contracts that they no longer need any on-the-spot help. But though the hospital's attorney is not present, you may be certain that he reviews all decisions as a matter of course. Similarly, although the experienced medical director may dispense with his own attorney during face-to-face negotiations, he can never dispense with his attorney's scrutiny of the contract prior to its final signature.

It is important in your conduct of all business matters to take appropriate notes, even during so apparently minor a contact as a telephone conversation. Most attorneys keep records of their meetings just as you keep records of all your contacts with patients in the progress notes. The reasons are similar. In both cases memory is very unreliable, particularly because future events can be so unpredictable. If you wish to have a telephone conversation with your attorney about a certain matter and there is sufficient time, you can mail him a copy of your notes and questions prior to calling him. If there is not enough time, you can make notes of the conversation and subsequently mail a copy to him so that there can be a follow-up. In either case you must build up a file of notes so that later you can establish that any material in question was discussed.

If you wait until you are in trouble before you start keeping records, you may find in court your absence of records is tremendously detrimental to your case. You may be certain that everyone with any legal or administrative training will have kept appropriate notes. An additional necessity for note taking, which you share with your attorney, is the subsequent step, namely, developing a checklist of items to discuss prior to any formal or informal meetings.

THE PRECONTRACT SURVEY

Almost as essential as having a legal adviser scrutinize the contract before signing is the necessity for a detailed, in depth, precontract survey of the department. You must personally inspect the premises, personnel, and any peculiar arrangements that relate to your department's activities. It is important to make this inspection when your negotiating position is still strong, that is, prior to the time you have signed an agreement. Once a binding agreement has been signed, everything that is not included becomes evanescent, no matter how important it may become to you subsequently. Thus unless you have taken the precaution of putting

into the agreement all of the elements that are essential to the performance of your duties, you may find yourself very quickly frustrated by gaps in memory or actual change in administration. You
must always bear in mind the possibility that the person with
whom you are now negotiating is not the person with whom you
made the initial agreement.

The hospital's attorney will scrutinize every provision in your
agreement; his duty is to insure that the hospital is not put to a
disadvantage. Therefore, as a matter of course, the contract will
elaborate at length upon your obligations to the hospital but keep
to a minimum the specification of the hospital's obligation to you.
Now if all you need to perform your duties is paper and pencil,
you may relax. But if you do require now or will in the future
require unusual equipment, a different configuration of department
space, or employees with specific talents that are not presently
available and if you have promised to perform functions that require one or more of those elements, then you had best be very
wary if the contract only specifies your obligations and fails to
mention these necessary elements as well.

When a missing element, be it space, equipment, or personnel,
will significantly affect department earnings, you may reasonably
expect that it will be provided as soon as practicable. However,
deficiencies that diminish the reputation of the department rather
than its earnings have less priority and will not be remedied unless
specifically identified and dated at the time of the agreement. Since
the hospital will expect you to deliver the services that you have
promised, you must be certain that you have all you need to
make delivery.

As an example, if the hospital promises you more room for
needed services but the present area cannot be expanded without a
major capital expenditure, you had best have that noted in an
amendment to the contract. Unless there is some sort of pressure
on the hospital to discharge its obligations to you, administration
may balk at doing so. This is particularly important if you know
that several other departments are being established at the same
time and that all of them will also require significant capital expen-

diture. You must have your dibs in writing or you may have to wait far longer than you would have expected.

The only ones who will suffer if (in the absence of documentation) the hospital should postpone delivery of obligated update, will be you and the patients your department should be serving. You may be reasonably certain that the administrator, responding to complaints generated by you, will skillfully point out to one and all that the hospital has given you everything that you have asked for on paper and that, as a first-class talent, you should be able to manage with what you've got.

If the contract you sign includes the proviso that your standard of performance is predicated upon the hospital's standard of backup facilities, then the black mark of substandard departmental performance will fall where it belongs, namely, on the administration. Second, most hospital administrators will try very vigorously to avoid promises, particularly of the blank-check type, and will instead demand a list of specific needs from you. There is more than a little element of trickery in the request; for administrators know by experience that no one can anticipate all of his future needs accurately or be able to list them in advance. If you are too specific, you may actually tie yourself down by asking for items that will not be appropriate when the time comes. So you must be as wary as they in detailing the resources you expect you will need.

Although it may appear otherwise at times, you and the hospital are not really in an adversary position. The problem is merely that most directors want more than they can properly utilize and hospital administrators rarely have the resources to provide all that the medical directors would like. You will have to be prepared for some bargaining and horse-trading, particularly if a similar type of negotiation is going on, or is about to go on, in another department. The precontract survey is in a way a trial of strength and political skills between you and the administrator. It is also an opportunity to further your relations with the medical staff by developing priorities for what they will need when you circulate your preliminary report—the precontract survey.

You had best, however, be circumspect in your use of the medical staff as a lever in your negotiations. Certainly if the administration balks at providing an essential service to correct some very obvious and glaring deficiency, you may have to resort to additional pressure from the medical staff. But it had better be a major deficiency, not merely the frosting on the cake. Recommendations set forth in the appropriate, logical manner will impress the medical staff. They can appreciate planning and goal-oriented problem solving and will look favorably on the fact that you have more on the ball then mere technical competence.

STANDARD DETAILS OF THE CONTRACT

Two model contracts from the Board of Medical Examiners of the State of California are shown in the Appendixes. They were drawn up for the guidance of physicians in radiology and pathology who wish to establish a contractual relationship with a hospital. Regardless of your specialty, you will find it worthwhile to study them closely to see what an official body regards as the vital elements of the physician-hospital contractual relationship.

Now as to the source of your specific contract. If you are a pathologist or a radiologist, you may be certain that the hospital already possesses a format for establishing a contractual relationship approved by its legal council and governing board. There are certain state and federal third-party payers that also may be used as a source of details of the contractual relationship. Most commonly, the hospital has its own standard contract (drawn up by its attorney) that it will present to the prospective medical director for his approval. The contract sets forth the basic components of the agreement. You will have to write in any unique and specific relations that also must be established.

Alternatively, the administration may suggest that the medical director and his attorney draw up a contract that the hospital will then process through its legal department for final format. Here, of course, the ploy may be that you will leave out some important elements. A fourth source of a contract detail is simply a written version of your final verbal agreements as to how the relationship will be established and maintained and how remuneration will be paid but leaving virtually all else unwritten or stated only in the vaguest of forms. This type of contract is the most dangerous, since often what is not written is more important than what is. Because these informal contracts rarely go into detail about anything except remuneration, they leave the medical director at the mercy of any subsequent memory lapses that the administrator may have.

Most contracts open with a general statement of the purpose and nature of the agreement. The preamble is important because it is here you will first see an outline of duties that you may not recognize or even acknowledge. The contract then specifically identifies the parties to the agreement and their legal addresses for purposes of documentation.

The contract must include a clear statement of the physician's status as an independent medical contractor. Since, by law, only physicians are legally entitled to practice medicine, your activities specifically as a practitioner of medicine are your own business and not that of the institution. Because the hospital cannot legally control your behavior as a practitioner of medicine, it cannot be held responsible for any acts arising from that behavior if it awards you the independent contractor status. That statement is especially important if you are to be a clinical specialist as well as a director of a department.

The matter is not quite so simple if you are a salaried employee. In that case the hospital's obligation to you is more extensive, since it does, in fact, agree to cover you completely, except for any acts violating the Criminal Code, and so must provide you with liability protection. Even here, though, the physician may be named as a specific defendant in a legal action because of some patient activity he has undertaken. The price of this protection is that the hospital can significantly limit the physician's activities in ways that he might not normally choose himself.

In this malpractice-oriented era, every contract provides that the physician-director will carry such professional liability insurance as is commensurate with his position and responsibilities. Furthermore, the agreement requires that he will present to the hospital legal evidence of the current status of his coverage and that, should he fail to do so, the hospital will provide the necessary coverage at his expense. Thus the hospital-based physician has a contractual obligation to maintain liability insurance that specifically lists him as an individual separate from the hospital. That may or may not accord with medical staff policy, since the hospital's bylaws may not require the medical staff to have insurance. The thrust of the action is to remove the hospital from risk when the medical director acts within the guidelines of his training and according to his conscience.

Negotiating compensation and financial agreements is so individually unique an activity that few useful general remarks on the subject can be made. Percentage standards vary widely with the nature of the service and the degree of the clinical and nonclinical involvement. Percent of the gross ranges from as low as 2½ to as high as 40. Arrangements based on the net are now so rare that not even a range can be quoted. The physician is advised, if at all possible, to contact his colleagues in the area to find out what percents are current there. Other hospital departments may also have percents that they will reveal, and possibly even some of the societies will have guidelines as to acceptable rates of remuneration.

Although most administrators have had no formal legal training, all have had extensive formal and informal training as well as extensive job experience in contractual negotiations. The man sitting across from you and talking about how much he is going to give you is not as innocent of the various nuances as he may appear; and if his long-range plans do not coincide with yours, you may find many entrapments in the agreement you negotiate. One of the administrator's major strengths is the tendency of hospital-based physicians to keep all details of the agreement secret.

The physician's assumption that he can keep his arrangements secret is somewhat ill-based, since obviously everybody in the accounting office knows the amounts of the checks and certainly the doctor's own office staff knows the details of his agreement. Nevertheless, it is administratively useful to keep the various medical directors divided in this area, since it is easier to negotiate with each individually. It is easy for the administration to imply that your arrangement is better than most, and so you tend to protect yourself by not letting anyone else know about your sweet deal.

In fourteen years of medical direction, I know of only two instances in which a physician spontaneously brought up the subject of his percentage, and in both cases it was to complain about downward revision at the last negotiation. Even when a physician is negotiating a retainer or salary type of compensation rather than a percentage, he must be careful about the method of remuneration, particularly in connection with the problem of growth. Failure to anticipate that problem can financially strain the physician and can even inhibit departmental growth, since help may become unobtainable. One physician in that predicament recently complained that he wished he had tied his salary, which was based upon the number of hours he worked for the hospital each day, to the hospital's room rate. Had he done so, he calculates he would be receiving enough additional income that (1) he could afford an assistant medical director and (2) he would not himself be so badly hurt by inflation. As it is, he is vainly trying to cope with a position that really requires two men.

The advantage of a salary or a retainer is that income at the time of the initial agreement is always more than adequate because it is not based upon departmental activity; consequently—and importantly to the administrator—the physician does not have to search for supplementary income. The physician who does not need to develop other income sources can devote his full attention to the hospital's department activities. You may be sure that the administrator also recognizes that, because of inflation, he will soon be paying the salary with less valuable dollars. On the other hand, you, as time passes and experience grows, give increasingly more valuable services in the same time span.

The model contract deals only sketchily with the administrator's responsibilities to the director in the operation of his department. There are a large number of minor but essential points that the director must specify if he is to have the full range of administrative authority to manage a department. Thus, if the medical director wishes to review each hospital staff member hired or if he wishes to review every change in job status and salary change, the contract must so specify. Similarly, only an explicit statement in the contract can guarantee him access to the financial records of his department. If he is not legally entitled to be informed of the financial details, he will never know the total situation and his planning will be distorted accordingly. Almost uniformly, administrators seek to withhold that information; for they have learned that power resides in the controller of information. In other areas, the director's authority may be bounded quite severely by the provisions of prevailing legislation, most specifically his authority to terminate and summarily dismiss employees. A contractual statement to the contrary will have no validity in that situation.

If you engage in any clinical activities, your contract should include a note on how to handle a conflict of interest. As we have already said, a conflict of interest becomes very insidious unless there is some established way to deal with it. An informal approach to the situation may be all that is required; but if you should find yourself in an adversary situation, you will thank the day when you had the foresight to draw up an outline of just how the matter would be processed.

OBTAINING AN ASSOCIATE

Every staff member must obviously be acceptable to a credentials committee and to the executive medical staff of the hospital. However, once these requirements have been met, nothing should hinder your integrating an associate into departmental activities. But in order to avoid further obstacles, your contract must include a statement of your right to get an assistant and your right to delegate all of the activities that you feel can be delegated. Otherwise, administrators can refuse to deal with anyone but you, the original medical director, and thereby functionally veto your choice of assistant. The administrator can even have his middle-management people do the same thing. They may put all the calls through to you, dump all the load on you, and, in effect, try to break the new associate by a process akin to Coventry.

You will find that process very disturbing, particularly if the department requires close teamwork of two or more physicians. You need explicit statements in your contract as to who will be the ultimate judge of what the associate does, what responsibilities he undertakes, and the method of handling decisions. Legally, if this associate is retained by you, then you are indeed totally responsible for his activities no matter what his medical competence as you see it. When there is a dispute over his activities, and you refuse to intervene, you may find such a mechanism as Coventry being used.

The problem lies in the different viewpoints between the medical director and the administrator; the administrator can reasonably expect the same degree of competence in the field of human relations as in the field of medical techniques. Most disputes about associates have arisen in the former area. A major problem at all levels has its origin in the following maladaptive human behavior trait: The more egotistical a person is the less effectively he can plan for the time when he will no longer be present to direct activities. That applies specifically to the agreements worked out with a dominant administrator who states that certain things need not be put into the contract because they can be handled on a one-to-one basis. Since this administrator is no less human than any other, he may retire, fall ill, become disabled, or even be terminated, whereupon the verbal agreements are nullified. You may be certain that whoever replaces him will be very suspicious about reputed verbal agreements in your favor reported to him only by you.

Thus you cannot rely upon anyone being at the hospital as long as you are, and that must be reflected in the provisions of the contract. Now, the reverse does not apply; the contract is quite explicit about what happens if you are no longer available. Certainly the hospital is not bound by any agreement you have made with an associate unless he is included in the contract at a future revision.

In those instances in which the administrator obdurately refuses to include provisions in the contract that are in daily use, you do have some other means of establishing the existence and validity of those agreements. However, the total burden of the proof is upon you. You must keep documented memoranda as to the areas in which you perform specific activities that are allowed and accepted by administration. A diary of such activities in which administration allowed you to act in a certain fashion for a prolonged period of time is useful only if it documents objective actions, consequences, and other data. Your mode or style of management is almost impossible to record. The more informal that is, the less useful it will be as a precedent when challenged. If all else fails, you may wish to outline your activities in the form of a letter written to the administrator. You should have evidence that he has received it, even though he refuses to acknowledge or otherwise imply assent. Certainly if he objects, he should register his objection in the same written form and you should have a copy.

Every contract must contain provisions for termination of the agreement and for adjudication of disputes. Obviously those provisions must accord with the basic hospital and medical staff bylaws. In most instances, the medical executive committee must be informed of any termination or contractual change. That is particularly important because there must exist some sort of advise-and-consent mechanism to give the medical staff input in the choice of the department head. In many institutions the director is selected by the administrator and other interested parties and is presented to the medical staff as a *fait accompli*; usually the medical staff merely rubberstamps the choice. Occasionally there are rebellions by the staff, but most hospital administrators are astute enough to defuse the conflict by whatever political means seem most appropriate to the occasion.

What this means to you personally is that in case of a major disagreement between you and the hospital in which the hospital has a valid objective point of difference, you as director may really have very little chance to hold onto your position. Even going to the medical executive with political support may be ineffectual if the discrepancy is a violation of your contract. Thus the legal agreement on the medical staff adjudication will be of use to you in your protection and security only when the contractual obligations are not in violation.

LIVING WITH YOUR AGREEMENT

Once you have negotiated each particular section and item, dotted each i and crossed each t, you must look at the entire package to be certain that (1) it is reasonable and its provisions can be fulfilled by both parties, (2) it can pass scrutiny by the Board of Medical Examiners of the state in which you practice, unless, of course, it is strictly a salaried arrangement, and (3) the medical staff agrees with the provisions in terms of your functions and obligations and the obligations of the hospital to you.

You cannot afford to fool yourself by accepting an unworkable agreement simply because you have already committed yourself. If you have already settled in that area and need desperately to stay, you had better be certain that the total Gestalt is correct. It is rare that you have no other options; you theoretically can always find some temporizing measures if even one of the provisions of the agreement is not acceptable. Unless you have all of your assets in liquid form and can move very easily on a week's or month's notice, you would be foolish to accept anything that is unfair or inadequate.

If you continue to work under unhappy circumstances, you may find yourself trapped into arrangements that will remove your freedom of action and sour your enjoyment of life. A chronic grinding situation is conducive to strong negative emotions, emotional exhaustion, and irrational responses to special circumstances, all of which are likely to result in even further trouble for yourself. Thus, if the agreement is not satisfactory and you cannot get its provisions changed, drop the negotiations. Never compromise the basic principles and essentials that you have established with your attorney and with your family.

COMMON PROBLEMS

Most contracts avoid dealing with certain problems that will ultimately come back to haunt you. The first of these problems is your access to the details of the overall financial performance of your department so that you may indeed plan for the future in an appropriate manner. The second is your involvement with and input to the departmental budgeting and budget-deciding procedure. That has to be on a wider basis than merely your own department. Many long-range plans for growth have floundered because of administrative secrecy about finances and future trends in contiguous areas.

The administration commonly keeps details of the activities of all other departments secret even though the others are presumably to share the same capital pie. In such cases you find yourself fighting, not the administrator, but your peers for a small bit of capital; administrators often promote that on the principle of divide and conquer.

A third problem has to do with the hospital's basic philosophy and the need to conform to certain standards of behavior or approaches to problems. If these were openly stated, you might find you could not conform to them. They are likely to involve emotions. Consequently, although trivial in terms of service provided, the issues are highly important because major conflicts arise when emotions are unbridled. The inclusions may be race, religion, creed, pricing policy, and even political affiliation.

Although you and the institution have agreed to work jointly toward a common goal, you have agreed to use and be used by each other in a manner set forth in the contract. If the administration has secret plans for using you in a manner contrary to your long-term goals, you certainly need to know about it.

The administrator may recognize your talents in other areas and try to push you into activities that are more in his interests than yours. If, in this regard, the administrator provides you with only a small retainer that is inadequate for your total support, he thereby implicitly acknowledges that he has not contracted for your exclusive services. However, he may never recognize that openly and may press you to enlarge your activities at the hospital in a manner that is not compatible with your goals or future plans. Of course, he can terminate your agreement if you will not give in and either renegotiate on his terms or find someone who will do what he wants. However, if you are so valuable to him that he must have all of your time, then he is not likely to let go of you for fear you will merely move next door and either set up a competing shop or enlarge the operation there.

ADHESION CONTRACT

There is a whole code of law about contractual relations between parties in a superior and inferior position. The common example is the contractual agreement between a father and a son who works for him. The son is clearly in an inferior position and may easily have his rights violated as a consequence. The same is true of a medical director entering into a major agreement with an institution. He may actually be coerced by an unscrupulous and astute administrator into accepting arrangements that are prejudicial to his own personal and professional long-term interest. His only protection lies in the provisions of the contract that stipulate just how far the administration can push him.

In most instances, however, the administrator has the ultimate weapon in this adhesion arrangement; he can allow the contract to expire, refuse to renew it, and then start negotiating again for an even greater position of strength. The ploy is most effective when the medical director has already established and committed himself by economic ties to the community. His ace in the hole may be active support by the medical executive committee, but only if he has unequivocally established the value of his medical and human relations service with the medical staff. All of this involves real eyeball-to-eyeball confrontation that the medical director is advised to avoid at almost any cost.

8
AVAILABLE PRACTICE OPTIONS

PRESENT AND FUTURE CONSIDERATIONS

Obviously, the practice options available to you will be determined by your specialty and by the particular position that is open to you. Within those limits, however, exist a tremendous number of variables that will be of paramount importance in the future if not at this time. Unless the position you are considering is clearly a transitory one, you should study all the nuances associated with the offer, both those stated and those implied or hidden. Whether you are in a purely diagnostic specialty or in one more clinically oriented, there will be potential variations in the position that you can manipulate by your own actions.

Most hospital-based physicians, for example, seek to develop their positions in such a way as to give them the broadest financial base. Whether that tendency is due to caution, desire for additional revenue, an interest in long-term expansion, or an interest in getting help in the future is of little consequence. The fundamental motivation is to increase your freedom of action in determining your future. You may, of course, choose not to bargain for additional options for a variety of reasons ranging from personal inclination to being faced with a fixed rigid contract on a take-it-or-leave-it basis. Take-it-or-leave-it offers are usually predicated upon competing talent being available for the position. That, however, is no argument against expanding your stability and financial base to whatever extent is possible.

After ten or twenty years of faithful service, you as the hospital-based physician will walk away with whatever you have in your pockets and your savings account. In that same time, a primary physician will have established an office and built up a practice and inumerable assets to sell or barter away. What you need to do is develop something that will compensate for that lack of financial stake in your future. The need, of course, is more pressing upon physicians with the status of an independent contractor than on those who take salaried positions that ultimately should give them tenure and job security.

The specialty physician with both diagnostic and therapeutic modalities has far more options than his purely diagnostic colleague. In addition to the departmental position, he may have some of the following alternatives:

1. Seeing patients as a teaching function of the departmental activity.
2. Seeing patients as a part of the therapeutic activity of the department in the form of departmental consultations.
3. Seeing patients outside of departmental activity in either a diagnostic or therapeutic capacity. In either case, a fee for service will be generated.
4. Seeing and following patients within and outside the hospital and providing long-term care as a variant of a primary physician.
5. Seeing patients under some form of retainer for another group of physicians.

The potential income from such activity depends, of course, upon your arrangements with the hospital and, more importantly, upon your ability to generate a demand and satisfy such a demand. As a junior associate your choice may already have been made for you;

you may be assigned either to purely departmental activities with no patient care, or to the exact reverse, or to a mix. The important point is whether the financial agreement you have made with your employer allows you to reap benefits from the extra effort you will be making. The following generalities relate to the extent of your freedom of action in local circumstances.

THE EGO NEED

As department head or as the accredited associate you undoubtedly will feel the necessity to prove, at every opportunity, that you can supply better patient care in your area of expertise than anyone else at that hospital. That may be a very laudatory endeavor if your prime function is to provide patient care on a fee-for-service basis. If your function is to manage the department, however, then frenetic activity may be counterproductive both immediately and over the long term. From that point of view, you must determine in advance how you will respond to the various emergencies that will very likely present themselves. Your choice should be influenced by your agreement with your employer and by the source of your income.

DETERMINING PRIORITIES

The manner in which you allocate your time is a fair reflection of what you regard as your primary loyalties. The simplest way to determine what those loyalties should be is to ask what you are being paid for. If the major portion of your income derives from departmental management activities, then obviously those activities should have the first priority and the greatest time allocation. If instead the major portion of your income comes from patient activities—fee-for-service or equivalent—you must tailor your approach accordingly. You need to answer the question fairly quickly so you can plan appropriately and establish the pattern of professional services that you will provide.

If you happen to have an in-between situation in which the sums for directing a department are limited but it is implied that you will make up for that with patient care, then you will immediately have a dilemma in establishing your primary loyalty. The hospital that wishes to pare its cost by paying the director minimal fees for his services really ought not to expect his unswerving dedication to its goals. Such a situation may tempt you to utilize the department to expand your clinical activities until clear conflict of interest arises.

That might actually serve the hospital's purpose, since bringing in a new physician—you—also brings in new patients. But be wary of the approach, because it may be only a temporary subsidy that will be dropped once you have established yourself financially and developed permanent hospital affiliations. If those are the implications, you should quickly ascertain whether the tactic has been used on other physicians. If it has, does there still exist a market for your clinical activities, or have your predecessors soaked up all of the patients in that area of specialty? In the latter case you could be in a dilemma with inadequate departmental income and inadequate patient fee-for-service income. This tactic is rarely discussed openly but nevertheless is used repeatedly.

OTHER OPTIONS AVAILABLE

Your personal lifestyle and long-term goals must be the ultimate consideration in selecting a practice option. There are a multitude of ways in every specialty to achieve a satisfying life with security, adequate income, and good retirement prospects. Some routes arrive more directly than others at one or more of the requirements; some may be detours or blind alleys, particularly if you are not aware of their implications. You may have temporary opportunities to make large amounts of money; but unless that is your only criterion for long-term success, some of your other needs may be left unfulfilled. The discussion here is offered primarily to physicians who now have or will have the opportunity to be directors of departments. For those who are assistants at present, however, the following remarks may be of some use in determining the type of assistant you wish to be.

As a department head with a clinical specialty you will have the following basic options:

— You act as a primary physician with the management of the department as a sideline.

— You act primarily as the director of the department with clinical or consultant activities.

— You are actually number one but pretend to be number two.

— You are a 9:00-to-5:00 hospital employee with limited responsibility in the clinical areas.

There exist numerous variations on these themes, each with its own positive and negative aspects. One is that you merely use the department as a stepping-stone into a practice. That has much to recommend it particularly if you can manage to hold onto the department and use it in your future plans. Establishing a department and using it to build up your practice means, of course, that your primary loyalties are directed toward patient care. Accordingly, you may become so busy that your management of the department will wither away, at which point you have several alternatives. They depend upon the professional and personal relations you have established at the hospital.

Ideally, you can utilize the departmental position as a place to try out potential assistants or associates before you absorb them into your clinical activities. Alternatively, you can let the administrator and the medical executive bring in someone who might or might not fit in with your long-term plans. Choice of the right course requires rapid estimation of the area's potential for establishing a large practice. If the demand is too small, you may find yourself trapped with not enough income from either activity. If there is no one in your specialty in that area, you may assume that the sky is the limit unless, of course, you are in a very limited specialty field.

As an independent contractor, the more you do for the hospital the more you receive, so that there is no question of where your loyalty lies. In this instance, the clinical load is acceptable; for it is merely another source of income that may be useful in the future, if developed, as a means of supporting another man.

The third option is something of a trap. If you pretend that your loyalty is with the hospital but go about building up a primary practice, you will generate resentment that is due to the hiatus between what you say and what you do. When you are in open competition, people can understand certain actions; but when you say you are not in competition yet act competitively, you cause negative reactions. If your manner of handling such conflicts promotes even further resentment, you will find it difficult even to be accepted as a department head, particularly if there are others in the community with similar subspecialty training.

The fourth option provides the immediate assurance of an adequate income as well as a lid on your clinical responsibilities. It is nevertheless a potentially troublesome choice if you are both therapeutically inclined and a type A personality. At the outset you will have very little to do, and you may find yourself gradually straying more and more to the clinical field to fill up the time. As you begin to act increasingly like a resident physician, the medical staff will recognize it and take advantage of you. Later, when your departmental duties grow more demanding, there will be pressures on you to maintain your clinical activities. At this point you may either work longer hours at fulfilling the clinical responsibilities than you had planned or, by denying the requests for clinical help, build resentment among the staff who have heretofore supported you.

CHANGING YOUR MIND

If you begin your directorship with a policy of providing help whenever it is needed but later restrict your activities, you will generate considerable resentment among the strong-minded physicians with whom you must work. The only way to avoid that undesirable change of mind is to begin with maximal restrictions upon your activities. Once that policy is accepted, you can ease up and begin performing additional services. Even with a 9:00-to-5:00 position, you will still have to spend additional time attending meetings and taking care of departmental affairs. If to maintain relations with the staff you also work additional hours doing clinical work, you may, over the short term, keep many staff members happy. Over the long term, however, you will embitter yourself or your family and thereby reduce your effectiveness.

MEDICAL STAFF PRESSURES

The medical staff expects every doctor to act the part, that is, to see patients and take care of them. The expectation is generated in part by the physician's selfish desire not to be troubled with special problems in which he is not particularly interested. If you are skilled in an area in which most physicians have little training or interest, you will encounter tremendous peer pressure to take care of patients whose problems, although not necessarily complicated, are less acceptable to the patient's regular physician. That type of pressure will be unrelenting and will persist for years. The only way to stop it is to give in and begin primary patient care. If that is not your long-term plan, you should be prepared to make no significant exceptions and resist the pressure for the same length of time—years.

FINANCIAL RULES OF THE GAME

One piece of information essential to the department head is that governmental bureaucracy has decided that each patient requires only one type of physician at a time. If you are consulting with the patient's primary physician on a complicated case, you will find that only your consultation and the first few visits will be paid for. That may take you quite a while to discover because of the lag time between delivery of service and payment by government agencies. By the time you do discover that not all your services will be paid for, the occasion is long past and no remedial measures can be taken.

All this creates additional pressure on you to take over primary care. If you push the other physician into the background and assume the primary responsibility, you will be paid for all the services you perform on that patient. So in addition to peer pressure, you will find financial pressures pushing you toward the practice of a wider, more general type of medicine than you had originally intended.

To reiterate, you will have to determine just where your primary loyalty lies. You may be certain that, whatever your choice, there will be pressure on you to go in the other direction, so it is best to have some clear idea of your long-term goals. Otherwise, you may easily become lost in a thicket of daily pressure. The confusion engendered will merely reduce your efficiency in all the areas that you had planned on servicing. To avoid the confusion, you should be aware of the two basic models of specialty patient care that are currently available in the United States today.

THE CONSULTANT—U.S. MODEL

The U.S. type of consultant is generally a physician who has had a subspecialty training but who conducts a general practice of internal medicine. His clientele include a smaller group of patients with illnesses in his realm of special interest. He will, however, assume the role of primary physician with virtually any patient. When a problem in his special sphere of interest is referred to him, he will take over the total management of the patient except for surgical problems, that is, he will manage not only the disease for which his expertise was requested but all other aspects of that patient's care as well.

The referring physician has no function apart from that of a casual onlooker and friend of the family. Since he is not running the case, his bills will no longer be honored and so he tends to disappear from the scene. The problems arise later on. By dropping off the case, the personal physician learns nothing about the subspecialty activities that prompted him to ask for help. When a similar case comes up, he is as perplexed as before and may have to seek help again. The U.S. type of consultant thus does not teach except in a formal teaching situation.

The other hazard is that if the subspecialist gets along well with the patient, he will almost certainly be asked by the patient and the family, because of his higher status, to take over the long-term management of the case. Since that is rather flattering, the consultant is likely to accede, and so the original physician will have permanently lost the patient. He obviously will not take the loss very kindly, particularly if he has been the prime physician for some time. Thus the primary physician is conditioned against asking for help because, each time he does, he loses control of the case and, more often than not, the case itself.

That scheme is perfectly satisfactory to the third-party payers, since it tends to keep their payments down in that specific case. Unfortunately, they are unable to see the long-term effects of such behavior, namely, that ultimately the primary physician will try to handle cases that are far beyond his expertise because he has been discouraged from asking for help. In the final analysis, it is the patient who pays for all of this by getting less than optimal help when he needs it.

THE CONSULTANT—EUROPEAN TRADITION

The European type of consultant sees the patient and works him up but then merely assists and supervises the primary physician in his ongoing care of the patient, provided the primary physician has the expertise and capability to perform the additional services with help from the sidelines. The consultant has only limited exposure on the chart since he is obviously not managing the case; only his initial visits will be honored by the third-party payers, so he is the one who makes the sacrifice. However, the primary physician does learn how to handle this type of case. He also learns that he does not lose his case, so he remains open to guidance from this type of consultant. As long as the consultant is subsidized, he can perform a one-to-one teaching function to the advantage of both physician and patient. What the physician learns may then be applied scores of times further, even at other hospitals, so the long-term beneficial effects are magnified.

The European approach to consulting will not burden the department head if consulting is only his sideline and his major interest is in and his income is from departmental activities. However, the financial burden does become onerous if he depends upon clinical activities to generate a significant portion of his income. Which consulting model he can adopt will therefore depend upon the managerial subsidy that the department head develops. If he is in a position to follow the European example, however, he will sometimes find that the primary care physician is very unhappy because what he really wants is to dump that case on someone else, and the consultant has effectively insulated himself from the demand of taking it off his hands. Additionally, in many cases, the family or the patient will want to transfer long-term care to the consultant and will not be able to understand why he will not go along. That, of course, may generate even further difficulties the outcome of which will depend upon the consultant's ability to handle human affairs problems.

CONFLICTS OF INTEREST

The primary physician who is only secondarily a director will be greatly tempted to utilize departmental resources to augment his clinical activities. The amount of attention and reaction that will attract will depend less upon his abuses of the system than upon the demand for his specialist services. If he is the only expert in his field in the community, the most flagrant conflicts of interest will bother no one. However, in communities in which a number of such specialists are in competition with each other, the cry of conflict of interest will arise at the first evidence that the department chairman is using his advantage to gain patients and fees for service income.

There are two principal ways the director actually can use his position to gain patients. The first is by preempting departmental resources so that his patients come first and his patient care is better than anybody else's. That enhances his reputation and thereby diverts the stream of clinical referral. The second method consists of department technical personnel actively promoting calling Doctor X for help whenever the situation seems a little bit sticky. Such open solicitations very quickly raise hackles. Since the other con sultant physicians provide an essential service to the hospital committee function on a voluntary basis, they will undoubtedly utilize the committee as a forum in which to raise their complaint.

There is no way a primary care physician with a busy office practice can compete effectively on a complex case with a doctor who is based in a hospital. Moreover, by being Johnny on the Spot, the man in the hospital can soak up every problem in his specialty area. Of course, if the department head is to move into an office-based posture, he will suffer from the same difficulties himself when someone else gains the advantage of the hospital position. That is more apt to happen when the director who moves into an office practice brings in an associate to handle the hospital; the associate may then use the very same technique on the director that the director had used on his peers. If there is any potential for division between them, a major rift may be inevitable. In that event the man in the hospital is in the superior position if he has any sense of human relations and political savvy.

DIAGNOSTIC SPECIALTY OPTIONS

Specialists, such as radiologists and pathologists, who have no direct patient care functions, still have the potential for setting up subsidiary activities. Most of them try to set up their operations in a large medical building. The only obstacle here is simple economics; is there enough volume for the operation to be profitable? The answer, of course, will depend largely upon the quantity of the competition in the area. If, as so often happens, the office building is next to the hospital, the specter of conflict of interest once again looms as the specialists divert outpatients from the hospital to their own offices. Obviously, the return on these services in their offices is by far greater.

You may be certain that the hospital will expect a good explanation. The problem can easily become sufficiently serious to lead to contract termination. One way to handle the situation is for the director to concentrate primarily upon his hospital department until those activities are booming. Since administrators are very conscious of labor costs, the director can point out that the outpatient volume, although only a small percentage, requires additional staff. It might, therefore, be cheaper to let the overload go elsewhere. Whether such a ploy can be sold depends upon the man and the circumstances.

SETTING UP AN OFFICE

Whether your interests are both diagnostic and clinical or clinical only, you eventually face the task of setting up an office. The primary care physician must have an office immediately, since that is where his major income-producing activities will originate, but all others can drag their feet and try to ascertain the financial prospects before they take the step. It is in fact advisable to do without for a while, just to see how necessary and effective an office would be for you.

Unfortunately, many doctors feel a kind of compulsion to have an independent area, paid for by themselves, with their own name on the door. If your potential volume is only two or three patients a week, plainly it would be foolish to indulge that quickly in ego gratification. But an acceptable and logical stopgap alternative does exist. If it is follow-up care you must provide, you can use your hospital's outpatient care department. That is not ideal, but it is workable over a short-term period. If you must in addition bill for services, you can either utilize a home office and the talents of your family or make an arrangement with a bank or other financial institution that offers a collection service.

But at some point you will undoubtedly succumb to various pressures and consider getting an office. If you need space for only a few hours a week, it may be best to begin by subleasing an office that is already staffed and equipped. Since the primary care physician usually works in excess of forty hours per week, he has evolved the custom of taking off one or more half days a week from his office on a regular basis. During those hours the office remains equipped and staffed and the space is useless to the physician. If you can find a group, so that more than one afternoon per week is open, you have a low-cost way of obtaining an office address with its facilities. If you can find several such groups, you can get an estimate from each one and choose the best deal.

All too often you will be approached by the man who was instrumental in bringing you to the hospital with the suggestion that you sublease his office. That rewards him for his efforts on your part, establishes a close affiliation between you and him that he will use to his own advantage, and allows him to keep track of what you are doing. While you search for a better arrangement, you can reply that you are trying to establish the fair market price and that you want to find out what the opportunities are if you should need them for expanding from one to two or three afternoons per week. As a new physician, subleasing an already established medical office offers you a chance to learn some basic medical economics without having to pay through the nose each time you make a mistake.

The exact amount of office time that you require will vary with your activity. You may want a place merely to see the odd patient, write a few notes, and have a few letters typed; you may want an office where they will answer the phone, take messages outside the regular exchange hours, do the billing, and coordinate appointments for you. Obviously, the more comprehensive the services that you require the higher the unit cost.

The more extensive your involvement in the office the greater your opportunity to work with an established team of medical assistants who will educate you in office procedures. Spend time during those office half days with the staff to learn as much of medical politics and medical economics as you can; it may be your best opportunity to gain that kind of information. You will also have an opportunity to work with several types of people and ascertain the characteristics you want in your own office staff.

HAVING YOUR OWN OFFICE

If you have been subleasing, it is advisable to hire your own medical assistant before you start setting up your own office. The additional income you can earn by having the assistance of this person is far greater than the salary you will pay. There are a thousand and one things involved in setting up an office (getting a business license, having phones put in, advertising, paper supplies, stationery, medical equipment, and so on), and it is useful to have someone do most of the leg work for you. The girls you have been working with in the sublease situation can be invaluable in helping you screen applicants for your office position for two reasons. First, they will not be working with the office personnel they help select, so they can be fairly objective in their evaluation. Second, they may be able to help train your assistant in your peculiarities of operation.

Your selection of a medical assistant is a far more critical decision than your choice of an office. Your experience with the office staff in the sublease situation should give you a reasonably good idea of the type of person you are looking for. Undoubtedly you will also have learned that the office staff tried not only to educate you but also to program you to follow their own office procedures. You may have had quite a difficult time in convincing them that your own mode of operation is necessary to your specialty. So when you at last employ your own medical assistant, you must devote enough time and attention to train this person in how you wish the operation to be carried out.

In many cases, your assistant, in an effort to please everyone else and improve your reputation, will try to get you to handle any and every clinical demand that comes along. Once such a pattern is set, it is almost impossible to change it without bitterness on both sides. If you have made a mistake and allowed the office staff to set the pattern, which you now find onerous, it will be one long uphill fight. Thus, it is essential initially to devote the time to explain in detail—including writing down in itemized fashion everything that can possibly be written down—the procedures you want, the type of calls you want, how you want other calls handled, what you will take and what you will not take, and what you want deflected or diverted or stopped. Unless you are a masochist, you will take these precautionary steps at the onset to save the expense of future aggravation and suffering.

Since you can hire only one person at the beginning, you must expect that he or she will be totipotent. However, when you need additional medical assistants in the office, you may find that this person is incapable of delegating work. Unless you step in at once and redirect him or her, you will have a procession of temporary extra help coming through and leaving while your original assistant becomes more and more embittered from carrying the whole load. As the director of a department you should be expert in delegating and training to delegate and consequently expert in teaching even your own office help what should be done. If you can't do that in your office, you can hardly expect to perform adequately at the hospital.

OTHER NECESSITIES

Whether you are subleasing or setting up your own office, you will need to acquire the services of a bank. Obviously, not all banks and bank managers are alike. It is worthwhile to go around and meet a number of bank managers to find someone with whom you can establish an empathic association, and it is also worthwhile to check up on the activities of that particular branch to make certain that there are no problems that your associates are aware of. Quite obviously, as a physician, your own problem will not be getting money; it will be not overextending yourself. Certainly at this time you also need an accountant, if for no other reason than taxes.

These additional resources, together with your attorney, should provide sufficient backup help to investigate all nonmedical practice decisions in enough depth and detail to make satisfactory decisions. In fact, these gentlemen may be the first ones to alert you to problems at the hospital, since they may be able to recount comings and goings there that put some curious matters in a different light.

QUICK-SETTING PRECEDENTS

Many of the more successful people in this competitive society obey a simple maxim: Interpret the actions of others in the manner that is most conducive to one's own welfare. Thus your innocent reactions during the first days, weeks, and months of your directorship will haunt you if they are unwise. Those reactions often include the impulse to be a good guy that has you doing favors for certain prominent physicians in the early stages of your career.

You tell yourself that you have a lot of free time and that, when they know you have no more free time, the doctors will no longer ask you for unusual favors. But you are merely fooling yourself. No one will give up an advantage so easily. The service may consist of following a case, on a weekend while the primary doctor is away, that you saw when there really was no need for you to see that case at all. Or a physician may ask you to do consulting work on a case that only marginally is within your field of interest or to see a problem case in his office. These are not favors, they are entrapments. Those who elicit them are expert manipulators who set up a situation because they are looking for a free ride.

Consider the case of the Friday night consult. The primary physician is going away on the weekend, but he has no one to sign out to. So he asks you to do a consult and to follow up the case. He may casually mention that he will be out of town on the weekend, so do whatever you think necessary. If you do as he asks, you had better plan on being in town every weekend, because the word will spread quickly that you will handle weekend coverage at the cost of just another consultation fee which the physician does not pay. That is an especially valuable service for the physicians and surgeons who are so subspecialized that they have difficulty in finding adequate cross-coverage.

CHANGING YOUR SPOTS

The only way to change your precedent-established spots is to change the scenery. That means changing the hospital, the office, and the office staff and starting afresh somewhere else. That drastic remedy may be the only one that will suffice if you have become enmeshed too deeply in practice activities that you wish you had never undertaken. I have seen a number of physicians on the treadmill of unacceptable demand who have abruptly, and often with great financial liability, moved somewhere else. Quite obviously, if you stay and fight, you will be wading knee-deep through a current of bitterness for a long time. That will undoubtedly have an adverse effect upon the various subsidiary goals you had hoped to attain in the first years.

If you really must be a good guy, start out by announcing a highly structured and restricted type of service. Adhere to those restrictions in the face of all pressures until it is established in everyone's mind that that is your way of doing things. Later, at your leisure, you can let the barriers down one by one for very special cases, whereupon the doctors will be effusively grateful rather than accepting your help as their due. The only good way to change your spots is to start out with no spots at all and add them later as you need them.

SETTING LIMITS ON WHAT YOU WILL DO

Quite obviously, you cannot work 24 hours a day, 7 days a week, 52 weeks a year. So in addition to establishing local precedents, you must use forethought in planning what your limits are in setting those precedents. This is more than merely a matter of saying, "I will do A but not B"; this is looking at your entire approach to clinical care. If your ego demands that you write all of the orders on a difficult case because no one else knows what to do, then you are not merely expressing a philosophy but also setting a precedent. How can you write all the orders from Monday to Friday and then expect the primary care physician to turn up on

Saturday and Sunday and handle the case until you get back? If you berate the physician each Monday because the patient has gone downhill, at some point he will suggest that you stay over and write the orders seven days a week. Instead of having a willing backup, you will have hostile, grudging help. If that is your approach, you must set a limit to your income so you can quickly get help you will accept; otherwise, you had better lower your expectations of others to a level compatible with your anticipated lifestyle.

Whatever limits you set will plainly affect your family as well as yourself. Can your family tolerate your declining or canceling almost every joint invitation because of your urgent practice obligations? Initially it may be exciting "that Daddy is late because he has to save someone's life," but it soon becomes old hat. Once you and your family are on divergent courses because their requirements and yours are disparate, separation at some emotional level becomes almost inevitable. Thus your limits will be determined as much by your wife's and your children's needs and desires as by your own expectations. The implications of all interlocking relations must be considered so that choices initially made will not be abrasive in the future.

A number of other forces will undoubtedly influence your limit-setting, and the most major of them is the hospital itself. If your agreement requires 24 hours a day care, 7 days a week, then you have, for whatever reason, set a zero limit on your obligations. Perhaps you would have preferred a lesser level of obligation but the hospital, by means of financial pressure, gave you no option. If they demand that you provide coverage that is obviously not within any one man's capacity, they must honor the limit they have set by providing the resources with which to do the job. They cannot simultaneously restrict you with respect to finances or personnel and demand a maximal clinical performance level.

One satisfactory way to handle impossible limits is to recruit a local physician to provide some of the clinical backup, particularly with your coaching. You can train him to handle problems that are new to him, problems that normally you would be called upon to see. That may not be totally satisfactory in the long run if you really feel you need people with the same specialty training as your own. Thus your very assumption of the mantle of leadership defines some of the limits, since as leader you are responsible for whatever happens, even when you are not there. If that is not the type of obligation you desire, you had best choose a more limited type of assignment.

THE GROWTH FACTOR

When you are offered a position, you should consider the growth potential of both the hospital and the community. Factors you should specifically consider include the following:

— Is this the only hospital in the area, or are there other hospitals?
— Are the medical staffs commingled between hospitals, or does each hospital have its separate medical staff?
— What is the current economic status of the area, and what are the population trends?
— What are the specific climatic, educational, recreational, and retirement advantages of the area?
— What is the relative distribution by age and number of the population?
— What is the relative distribution by age and number of the medical staff with which you will be working?

An area with only one hospital is a far different situation in terms of growth potential than one with multiple hospitals vying for the same market. In the latter case dissatisfied medical staff can play musical chairs and cause tremendous economic backlash on the hospital-based physicians. On the West Coast, disgruntled physicians have actually moved out and established other hospitals so that the competition, instead of remaining the same or decreasing, has increased.

Economic prospects in an area are obviously a great concern, since the rate of return for different services varies with age and health plan coverage. Certainly an area that is expanding economically will have a far different capital outlay picture, as reflected in hospital budgets, than an area that is contracting. All this influences the ability of the area and yourself to attract additional help when it is needed.

The demographic distribution of hospitals, patients, and physicians may also be significant. With regard to the patients, the older the population the more recurrent utilization of services they will require. The older the medical staff the more difficult it will be for them to recruit associates; as one grows older, he grows less flexible and accommodating. When opportunities are available in many areas, an older associate is less appealing. So as long as there is no room for new primary physicians to move in directly, older physicians will tend to keep a lid on hospital utilization.

The medical director who has moved into an area that contains several hospitals, none of which have had adequate facilities in his field of expertise, has a very quick and sure way of determining how he is doing. If within six to twelve months after joining the staff at Hospital A he has not heard from Hospital B, C, or D, then he has cause to worry. That is particularly true if the other hospitals have no staff physicians with his skills. When a large hospital brings in a physician to establish a department, it is common practice for the peripheral hospitals to see if they can get a piece of him, that is, to gain access to services without having to invest a major sum of money in getting him into the area. Of course, that accessibility depends upon contract details. However, even if you have an exclusive contract with Hospital A, the fact that Hospital B, C, or D does not inquire into your availability should be a disquieting reflection on your public relations.

VERTICAL VERSUS HORIZONTAL GROWTH

Depending upon your specialty and your particular circumstances, you may have a choice between vertical and horizontal growth patterns. Vertical growth refers to an exclusive affiliation with one hospital at which departmental activities are growing more complex and numerous each year so that the total output grows at a very steep rate. Horizontal growth refers to a situation in which you gradually add other hospitals and associates to your sphere of control so that, again, total output grows at a very steep rate. Each situation has long- and short-term advantages and disadvantages that may be further complicated by the vagaries of the local circumstances.

In the case of vertical growth, you can concentrate all your attention on one institution. With all of your public relations efforts directed at one medical staff, you should rise to high planes of influence. You waste no time driving back and forth, and because you are at only one institution, you have a high degree of visibility there. The problem is that, if you are not altogether successful, your contract can be canceled or significantly adjusted. Moreover, since you have no other base of operation, the administration can exert far more pressure upon you and make you do their bidding in matters in which you might have chosen otherwise.

Even if you get along very well with the present administrator, the ravages of time may suddenly present you with a new man in the position of power and you will have to start all over again. New people may move in with new ideas and a new team roster, and you may find yourself shunted to the sidelines. Finally, if you have an unsatisfactory agreement with the administration, you may find it exceedingly difficult to get them to approve and fund an associate. If you already have an associate who subsequently splits from you over the usual problems of interpersonal relations, he likely will remain at that hospital and compete directly with you.

Horizontal growth has its own unique costs. First of all, it may clearly violate the original contract; you may add one only to lose one. Second, there may be so much antagonism among the various administrations or various medical staffs that, being no one's man, you are trusted by no one and so have less influence rather than more. Horizontal growth entails time wasted in traveling and reduces visibility, since you are divided among two or more institutions. Your influence with each of the staff will be reduced accordingly. If you have any primary patient care activity at all, you must look out for a further conflict of interest, since you may get patients from one hospital that subsequently are admitted to the other.

If you can overcome those difficulties, however, horizontal growth has some distinct advantages. If you have a number of talents that cannot be fully utilized at any one of the hospitals, you can spread them out over several hospitals. You may then take advantage of the competitive spirit among hospitals by setting up some unique segment of service in each department. The initial hospital may then adopt what it had originally turned down.

Administratively it is easier to manage small departments than large ones; as the number of staff increases arithmetically, the human relations problems increase exponentially. Your managerial capabilities will be less strained by two hospitals with staffs of fifteen than by one hospital with a staff of thirty. The greatest advantage of a second hospital is that, by expanding your financial base and by not being at the mercy of one administrator, you become more secure emotionally as well as professionally.

Your stronger position will make it correspondingly easier to get funds to hire help. It may even be an advantage in recruiting, since the physician you are wooing may feel that, if he can run one of the departments for you, he will have far greater independence than he would have were he merely to be your chief assistant in a big department. Whether or not you delegate a department to him is, of course, your own business. Following on that advantage, if there is a split, it may be that each of you will take a hospital. If the acrimony is not too great, it may be possible to maintain some sort of cross-coverage and working relationship, even though you are now both totally independent.

GETTING HELP

An outstanding characteristic of administrators is their penchant for authorizing additional help only when additional paperwork substantiates the need. Of course, the paperwork requires extra time just when you are busiest and most overworked.

If you had the time to do the paperwork, you probably would not require the help.

When someone else controls the purse strings, you can be sure that your load will have to go up well over your maximum capacity before he will even consider getting you an assistant. All too often, the chronically overworked physician tries to compensate by cutting back on areas in which reduced effort will not show. Plainly that response is not conducive to long-term ongoing quality care. Controlling your own purse strings is therefore one of the most important initial steps you can take. Even though the arrangement with the hospital gives you less money initially, the freedom it gives you downstream is usually worth the price.

The medical director who cannot directly budget monies under his control for recruiting an associate must begin the campaign for getting help far in advance of his actual need. He can anticipate that months or even years will pass before the request is approved and the need is met. That is particularly true of those specialties in which there are wide fluctuations in demand for services, so that the director is overloaded only for a substantial fraction of the year. By the time you have all your arguments wound up and ready to go, the demand begins to drop and the matter is postponed. Yet each time that happens you know that, had you been able to meet the demand with full services, the total of utilization might have continued climbing. As it is, demand drops back as people find they have to wait longer and longer.

If you are located in an area with access to training programs, find out how your prospective applicant performs under fire by trying him out on weekend or holiday coverage. (That procedure, of course, can be followed only when the funds are available to pay him and you can get the medical staff privileges as well as the malpractice coverage.) It may be possible to use the same approach with an older man in your field who wants extra work, but he will undoubtedly be burdened with far more family pressures and other limitations on his freedom of action. Those who are already established often restrict their relocation efforts to areas within a reasonable drive from their current place of residence. And indeed, many suitable applicants exclude themselves by refusing to move on a temporary trial basis.

Nevertheless, you cannot hire a man without trying him out; for neither you nor he receive any benefit if he joins you only to break up very quickly in an acrimonious dispute with distress on both sides. You must see the candidate in action in order to assess the intangibles that are so essential to a lasting relationship.

A good way to get temporary help is to locate someone in your specialty in practice in your community. He may wish to restrict his practice to your field of common interest and thus agree to cross-cover in exchange for some benefits that you must establish. He will probably extract as much advantage from you as you from him, since he will be as overloaded as you. If the two of you work out reasonably well together, you may be able to work up a position for a junior associate to help both of you in various ways. The principal difficulty here is the inevitable tendency for the younger man to side with one or the other of the two older men. Unless you are willing to work assiduously in maintaining a reasonable relationship, the arrangement can fracture relatively quickly.

SUBSIDIZING THE COMPETITION

In observing my colleagues over the years I have been amazed at the number who have, in effect, subsidized the very physicians who later became their most bitter competitors. The recurrent theme is that of Doctor A recruiting Doctor B as his assistant. Doctor A works at a tremendous pace to accumulate the funds to recruit someone and then brings in this young man with high expectations of less demand upon himself. Yet in one or two years they have dissolved their association and Doctor B is in practice openly competing with Doctor A.

The basic problem is that Doctor A did not set up a proper environment for a number-two man, one in which the relation could persist indefinitely. He may have been a loner who was impossible to work with except on a short-term basis; perhaps he was too egotistical and demanding, or maybe he was unable to stop competing with someone on his own team. An equal array of faults may have existed in the assistant. In any case, the reason for the final separation invariably is personality clashes, conflicts that, in theory at least, are always avoidable.

There are several options open to the doctor who feels betrayed because his one-time associate has become his competitor. Having a competitor in practice can in fact relieve you of a substantial amount of your clinical load if you have a departmental income as well. Thus you can actually use your competitor as a helper, even though he would not be happy to hear himself so described. Often the very reason the competitor is in practice is because he knows the delightful arrangement the original medical director had and hopes to have one just like it. The medical director therefore feels constrained to drive him out by starving him, and so they end up in a long and acrimonious struggle.

A partnership, medical or business, is much like a marriage. There is a courtship phase when both parties try to please each other, the initial legal relationship, and then, as the two parties no longer try to make allowances for each other, a development of suspicion, bitterness, acrimony, and a year or two later, open conflict. The only locale relatively immune to that syndrome is the civil service of a government institution in which everyone has salary and tenure. There the opportunity for local small group relationships does not exist.

Thus the first element in establishing a satisfactory, long-lasting relationship is to assess your ability to work with someone. If you really are a loner, you had better set up an arrangement in which both you and your potential helper are totally independent. If you take the time to question doctors who are in long-lasting relationships, you will be surprised at how many are working together for mutual advantage but remain financially independent of each other. Since their only commitment to one another is mutual help, they can coexist as long as neither one takes advantage of the other.

The second essential element in holding on to number two is that the work planned for him be rewarding enough that he will stay with the position. More often than not it isn't the money you pay, it is what you dump on him that creates the problem. You, as the founder of the department, presumably worked many long hours and were on call every day and every weekend. When your associate finally arrives and you dump all the call time on him, he will remember only his long hours, not yours, and he will immediately resent the advantage you take of him. If, however, you share the workload with him equally and in general share a reasonable portion of call time, he may, particularly if he has any chance for self-aggrandizement, work out a modus vivendi that will be long-lasting.

The third major ingredient in a successful association is competent legal advice. Very few papers need be signed in a marriage because there a long-standing contractual history and numerous subsidiary laws exist to handle problems at the time of a split. A partnership or an association does not have similar precedents. Therefore, you must write your own clauses for the honeymoon period, the subsequent period, and even for the period of separation. Your "marriage contract" may seem unnecessary when you are perfectly happy to live together; but when the time comes to split up the property and the family, you may wish you had something on paper.

The fourth critical element in all of this is the personal relation between yourself and number two. That goes much deeper than merely your interaction at work; it extends into your family, including especially the relation between your wives. If you unthinkingly assume that, because you like his work, you will like his style of living, and if you insist upon socializing, you may find that basic disagreements between your wife and his will accelerate any incipient split between you and him.

Wives of doctors are the least accustomed to dissembling and acting diplomatically of all of executives' wives. In business circles people are much more aware of the pecking order and are consequently much more circumspect in their behavior. Obviously, the senior vice president is more important than the junior vice president and the wives are aware of that and behave appropriately. In medicine, however, status is more often related to the type of specialist you are, whether you have your boards, and which school you graduated from, all of which may have nothing to do with your position in the pecking order at the hospital. Yet the wives react to the artificial pecking order. When a senior wife whose husband is not board-certified finds herself attacked by a junior wife, she quite naturally is annoyed.

Since in any case number two is usually on when you are off, and vice versa, there is really very little rationale for much socializing, particularly if you two have very different lifestyles. Socializing should be kept to the irreducible minimum that is just sufficient to show that you do speak to each other apart from work. Beyond that it can do nothing but provide an opportunity to ignite powder trains of emotional argument that may eventually lead to an explosion that will destroy the association.

ORGANIZING A GROUP

Your ambitions may not be satisfied merely by acquiring an associate; you may wish to set up an entire group. Whatever your reason, the consequence of the decision will be that your group will handle all the clinical work as well as the hospital work in the area. Obviously, you will then control all the income and share all the calls for services. This is a laudable plan if you have the stamina and the planning ability to carry it out, but you must be prepared to put in an inordinate amount of time.

One of the basic strictures of medical organization perceived by Neal Hamil, M.D., is that "he who administers ultimately leads." If you acquire not only a number two but also a number three, four, and five, there will arise a great deal of clerical and administrative work having to do with work schedules and record keeping and meeting with the office staff, the accountant, the lawyer, the administrator, and so on. If you begin delegating more and more of it to one of the junior men, you will have unconsciously and unwisely delegated the functions of leadership to a potential competitor. There is a phenomenon known as a palace revolution: the leader is deposed and a new leader from the ranks takes over. Often the only way the original leader can protect his investment is to break up the group and take the biggest pieces with him. But although the expedient has immediate survival value, its long-run effect is to put him back on square one.

It is very tempting to move into an area, develop it, bring in more and more assistants, and, once you have built all that up, take your reward by leaving most of the work to your juniors. Inevitably, however, the people you have brought in will recognize the disparity between what you do and what they do and between what you receive and what they receive. Your juniors will give you no consideration for the work you did before they arrived; they were not there to witness your long hours of labor. The absentee landlord of a medical group is in a precarious position in the event of a determined attack from within. Unless you have a tremendously superior ego and all your associates are type B, your association is in danger from the time you stop being visible and doing a fair share of the work.

DISASSOCIATING YOUR ASSOCIATE

When your associate becomes less and less a helper and more and more an obstructionist or a budding competitor, it may be wise to put aside some long-term goals for short-term advantages. If you can realize, prior to an open break, that he is a potential rival and that the more open the separation the more serious a rival he is, you might make far more compromises to keep him on your team; for as a team member you still retain at least partial control of him.

If you are unwilling to live in a state of armed truce, you must immediately begin planning to disassociate number two. The decision is based not on your personal likes or dislikes but merely on the pragmatic aspects of the situation. Hopefully you will have drawn up an agreement of collaboration prior to the formalization of your association. You must remember it is possible to draw up a satisfactory document of separation only when both parties are still on speaking terms. Now, whether you are the director looking for an associate or an associate looking for a post as associate director, it is of crucial importance that you have legally valid assurance of what will happen if and when the crunch should come. Gentleman's agreements are of no consequence when neither side regards the other as a gentleman.

Obviously, as a director, it is to your advantage to make a separation agreement as early in your affiliation as you can, since your position of dominance will then be most clearly apparent. Your associate is likely to accede to most of the measures you propose at that time. However, you will find that even your own attorney will give your associate far more separation benefits than you feel he deserves, and certainly far more than you would want to deliver when conflict is in full force. Even common-law marriage partners, at least in California, are entitled to fair shares when their association breaks up.

It may be that one partner was clearly dominant, did most of the developing, and generated most of the benefits, but the mere fact that he needed the help of another to achieve success establishes the importance of the other and consequently the other's right to his fair share. The document you draw up should act as insurance against a breakup, because your potential rival will be able to see just what he will get in comparison with what he might wish to get in the event of an open break without a contract.

If your long-term plan includes only the option of having someone work for you in a master-servant relationship, you had best change your associates at frequent intervals. However, you may find yourself developing a great personal liking for one of these associates. That is fine if during a long period of courtship you have worked out a stable modus operandi. That is probably the only way to prevent a partnership from dissolving—to keep someone on a temporary basis long enough to be sure of him. However, the duration must not be too long or again the association will turn sour.

If separation becomes necessary, one way to approach it is to keep the person in a subservient position and, at the first sign that you and he do not work readily together, start gradually restricting his degrees of freedom. You assign him work or duties that clearly do not meet his interests or desires and thus gradually squeeze him out by attrition. Since you continue to pay him even when he does less and less satisfying work, he will at some point, unless he is prepared to make an open break with you, merely start looking elsewhere. One day you will be happily surprised when he announces that he is leaving.

Another set of problems arises in connection with an associate who is very ego-dominant and who clearly has superior training and high expectations. Trouble is particularly apt to happen if he is obviously doing a major part of the work but is receiving a significantly smaller share of the income. At some point he is going to resent your advantages and begin plotting to take your deal away from you. Unless you have taken proper precautions to bulwark your position, particularly in areas where you might be vulnerable such as your status with the medical staff, he may just succeed. More commonly, he will make a major mistake in strategy by alerting you to his plans too soon. You can rush appropriate reinforcements to the point under attack; the palace revolution will fail; tempers will flare; and separation will take place very rapidly and bitterly.

If either during or after a separation you and your associate go around maligning each other, both of you merely end up losing respect among your peers. The common attitude that "if you use him, you are no longer my friend" presents a dilemma that the other staff physicians solve very neatly. Since if they use Physician A, they alienate Physician B, and vice versa, they use neither. I have seen that happen on numerous occasions. All of a sudden, during the course of an internecine struggle, departmental activity begins to drop and no one can understand why. Only years later does it become apparent that all the primary referring physicians were sending their cases to other hospitals because they had developed serious reservations about the effectiveness of people whose emotions ran so strong. That is something that emotionally involved people always miss. They notice it only later when the administrator of the hospital finds out about the matter and brings it back to where it began.

There is only one way to disassociate an associate with a reasonably happy result, and that is to use the horizontal growth technique. You establish departments at several hospitals; and each time you have an opportunity to pick up an associate, you give him one of the departments as his primary responsibility. When the time comes for the struggle and the separation, the new man will likely keep that department and then move out into his own area. Meanwhile your practice involvement will gradually restrict itself to the hospitals that you still manage.

Depending upon the amount of heat generated, the now independent entities may eventually be willing to work together again and share call. In the interim, while there is no actual sharing of call or even case load, there is another alternative for the director who is overburdened. He can mention the fact that there are other people in the area whom he brought in and that it might be useful to refer some cases to them, since he cannot carry the load alone. Thus you may have use of them—if they are indeed open for clinical work—even without being formally affiliated.

Finally, the director may find himself being squeezed out of his own base hospital. The problem may be that he is taking off too much time, his visibility has dropped to near zero, and his associate is doing all the work and taking all the credit. Consequently, he has lost the support and loyalty of his constituency, the medical staff. Even though he may have an adequate legal document to protect himself, his very absence from the hospital may invalidate it, since most such documents specify the extent of coverage required. However, the squeeze-out ploy requires the connivance and cooperation of the department supervisor as well as the administrator. The ploy is most likely to be attempted when there is a change of administration with a corresponding change in the tenor of the medical staff.

The medical director may now find the rules of the game changed considerably. He may, in effect, be removed from the game, since he no longer receives information and participates in no decisions and thus becomes a virtual nonentity. Finally, when contract renewal comes up, his contract is not renewed, and a new one is let out with someone else. This, of course, hardly seems like a fitting end for a chapter entitled Available Practice Options, but one of the practice options available is failure. Sometimes a roaring success contains within it seeds of a subsequent failure because of an inability to cope with the demands generated by initial success.

9
PLANNING
YOUR
FUTURE

YOUR GOALS

The hallmark of the truly effective manager is ability to plan a personal course as expertly as a departmental one. Now the fact that you have, or are well on the way to achieveing, a post of medical director implies that some form of long-range planning has been in operation. But after ten or twelve years of single-minded, dedicated effort toward a single goal, it would not be unusual to forsake further long-range planning and to say instead, "I've had enough of that, I'll just live the way I want to." But that response merely shifts the planning activities from the conscious to the unconscious level of your mind and so puts them beyond reach of logical input and decision.

In fact, no professional man with the responsibilities that you have can exist without setting and achieving a great many short- and long-term goals. In the business world that is called management by objectives. Of necessity you are already a charter member of the planning group and have, by your very successes, paid your dues. You may as well continue to take advantage of the skills that you have so painfully acquired over the preparatory portion of your career.

The moment you make a formal commitment by signing a contract, you have established some sort of two-, five-, and ten-year goals. A very few limit their goals to income alone. Rather, they imagine that they do; for it is inconceivable that income could realistically be a total goal. The majority of successful managers include other objectives, particularly the more intellectual ones that make man the distinctive creature that he is. To gain a clear sense of your long-term objectives, you need to ask, "Just what do I expect to be doing in ten and twenty years? Have I really chosen the right approach?" True, you may just follow your nose and hope to end up where you wanted to be; you may, that is, adopt the motto "All I ever wanted is what I've got!" However, unless you firmly adhere to the philosophy of predestination, you will want to devote considerable attention to the course of your future activities so that you remain the captain of your ship.

Chapter 8 detailed the tremendous variety in career options open to you. The problem is to choose the one approach most suited to your circumstances and most likely to satisfy your objectives. Of course, by choosing one alternative, you eliminate all others; and as time passes, it becomes increasingly difficult to change your course toward a radically different port. Some may try to surmount the difficulty by not choosing a goal at all, but in that way they rely totally upon capricious events to direct them toward a destination that they have to find acceptable.

In determining your objectives you must, of course, consider the desires of your marriage partner and your family. Most people with college and graduate school education expect from life a greater variety, challenge, and learning opportunity than those not so fortunately equipped. No doubt your spouse and your children will share those expectations. Thanks to modern preventive techniques and technology, it is now possible to lead a long, productive, and vigorous life, so both you and your spouse will probably have the opportunity to indulge in several careers if you so choose. Your choice now may determine whether you and she will be in a cul-de-sac thirty years hence or in an area in which numerous options are still open. The number of professional people who are trapped, by their own lack of planning, into work and lifestyles that they find onerous but by which they are held hostage through financial and other commitments is not small.

One way out may be the second-career approach. Because of the long-lived nature of physicians as a class, it is a reasonable alternative. With adequate planning, the multiple benefits of your position should put you in a situation in which you can change course if circumstances dictate or your interests change. Another reason for considering such an alternative is the press of scientific and technological change in the field of medicine. Whatever your speciality, if you examine its history, you will notice that it began by budding off from a more basic area. At times the offspring overshadows the parent. Such changes are still taking place and could occur in your field; in ten or twenty years you may not be doing what you are doing now because the situation has been so radically altered.

Additionally, you may anticipate such developments as the arrival upon the scene of young talent with newer skills and technologies. That will be of particular importance if you are situated in a hospital that is not in the mainstream of developments in your field. In that case, growth effects may at first be delayed and diffused and then occur precipitously, giving you very little time to accommodate to them. It is therefore obviously essential that you continue your present awareness of all of the significant trends in your field not only to maintain your technical competence but also to help you maintain your position.

Consider, for example, nuclear medicine. This relatively new and rare medical subspecialty overlaps both radiology and laboratory medicine, but even with that competition it is a promising and vital field of activity. Yet a new family of instruments heralded by the EMI scanner has now appeared on the horizon and may radically alter the entire field within a very few years. The responses that people in this field evolve to meet the new challenge bears very directly upon their own survival as a distinct class of subspecialists.

Indeed, this stands as a clear warning to all other specialties: they cannot consider themselves safe on the basis of current technology.

Another trend the impact of which may affect you personally runs counter to the decade-long schismatic evolution of smaller clinical subspecialty departments from larger departments. Due to changes in the population being served, there is increasing pressure for reintegration of those separate fields into larger multidiscipli-nary areas of activity too all-encompassing to be overseen by any one person. Your survival in the future may depend upon your becoming a member of a team instead of acting as team leader.

A far more obvious trend at this time is the personal conflict involved in the medical director's profession as a physician and his role as manager. As the small department he manages grows larger and larger by expansion of need and by his own services, he will find himself devoting more and more time to management and less and less to his professional activities. As the number of complex department services and the number of staff to supply such services increases arithmetically, he will notice that the number of machine-people and people-people interactions and problems goes up exponentially. The expansion of your human relations and management abilities entails almost by corollary a corresponding contraction of your medical specialty abilities. At some point you may suddenly realize that you will soon cease doctoring altogether, and that may bring changes in your self-esteem and in your peer relations.

Physicians are programmed, over the course of their training, to act independently; that has been a successful approach to the prob-lems we have faced. However, our value to society may shift in the future so that we will be useful only as small parts of larger teams because of radical demographic, technologic, and social changes that we neither appreciate nor wish to accept. Your very ac-ceptance or rejection of a pragmatic approach to your profession may determine whether you will be able to adapt your work and lifestyle to such changes. If you discern that you are not likely to adapt, an alternate career in a less rapidly changing environment may be your solution. In any event, it is apparent that some behavior patterns will have more survival value in the future than those you presently exhibit. The question you must answer is whether you will be able to adjust as circumstances change. In other words, what is your degree of manageability and adaptability under stress?

Consider the new medical director whose specialty is a field in which there is no formal training for the paramedical personnel he employs. He may choose a position that seems satisfactory to him only to find out that it involves far more on-the-job training and teaching than he is prepared to undertake. If he responds to personnel mistakes that arise from lack of training by blowing up, he may develop tremendous conflict, since those periods of stress will be recurrent. Thus he must radically alter his behavior in such a way that he can accept mistakes without exploding or suffer the consequences of continued severe psychophysiological stress.

When he finds himself in charge of five, ten, or fifteen people, all of whom require training, his behavior may actually become self-destructive. The management of a large number of personnel requires the capacity to adapt without emotionally overloading yourself at recurrent intervals. You can do that by withdrawing into the cul-de-sac of the role of the technical adviser, in which case you have less control over events, or by giving up the idea of working in such a team-orientated environment and retreating to the safety and insularity of a one-man practice. Even that last refuge, however, is subject to scrutiny by the government and third-party payers with their questions about indications, quality control, and utilization. In the final analysis it may be easier to change your attitudes than those of the society in which you live.

To put all this in another way, there must be some sort of harmony between what is required of you and what you can deliver. Certainly many will find they have chosen the wrong slot. To find out what you can do requires that you assess the resources available to you, and your primary resource is yourself. An honest evaluation of your qualities, including both your strengths and your deficiencies, is essential; for you must then compare your list with the description of the job to which you are actually or potentially committed. The realization that you may be faced with disaster if you persist in your present course may give you the courage to alter your present career radically in favor of something with far greater promise of long-lasting tranquility.

YOUR WORK

Once you have chosen a specific direction, you need to ascertain more details about your choice. Which will come first: your obsolescence, your disablement, or your retirement? The answer will depend upon how thoroughly you have prepared yourself for your line of endeavor and the events that occur once you are out in the actual work setting. You should be able to see trends in your specialty that are minor today but are likely to be major in another ten or twenty years. Was your training such that you can easily get in on the ground floor of the forthcoming changes, or will you have to take time off from the job to acquire the new techniques? If the latter, will you even have the time and opportunity to improve and upgrade yourself?

Here, then, is one matter of concern to all hospital-based physicians: the time to cope with new technological changes. In addition to such other pressures as peer expectation, there is growing evidence that bureaucratic pressures will require, for your future economic survival, more than a modicum of continuing medical education. When you consider the current public attention focused on quality and cost of care, on professional liability, and on the question of continuing competence, you have even further reason to assess your present qualifications seriously and to budget specific time for continuing medical education in the future.

Because of the position to which you have been appointed, it is obvious that the hospital's medical staff feel you can satisfy their needs. Satisfaction with your services, however, may not be a permanent fact of life. You may be certain that the staff will change as older men retire and newer men step in. Together with changes in technology, public awareness, and other factors presently unanticipated, that may radically alter the basis of evaluating your services.

In estimating the probability of your premature obsolescence you should take into account the accelerating trend away from reliance on results toward reliance on both results and the number of extra diplomas you may have. If you do not possess those extra plaques certifying your formal status as a specialist, you may be embarking upon a continual series of confrontations about your lack of "credentials." Not only will your peers, especially the younger men, expect you to be credentialed, but it is apparent that the bureaucracy may soon be differentiating among various skill levels by paying different rates. The professional societies in the Western World are currently in a ferment over paper-credentialing as a proof of capability. For all those reasons such credentials may be essential to survival in the post you hope to occupy for years to come. I have already seen several careers altered because of problems centered on this "lack of credentials." If you do not already have your boards, you should certainly make realistic plans to acquire them while that is still practical.

You may say, "Well, I can't acquire my boards now, so instead I'll obligate myself to a definite time allotment later for concentrated additional training." But unless such training is presently available in the time that you will allot to it, you are merely fooling yourself. The problem with such training is that attendance at most meetings, courses, and workshops is voluntary and signing in is no proof of attendance. And although informal credit may be gained, no formal credit toward any valid, widely recognized certification is presently attainable.

The most serious shortcoming of all is that these training courses are essentially book learning in which you hear about techniques rather than perform them. Few training institutions will allow you to work on their patient populations without having a chance to screen your initial stages of competence before advancing you to the level you desire. Thus this approach to on-the-job training for practical skills may be less than a reality for the majority. True, the various specialty societies are addressing this need to update practical skills in their workshops. Whether there is or will soon be adequate supplementary training in your field and whether you will be able to afford the time or the money to attend are, of course, open questions. One might add that the medical staff would be happier to see you, the resident expert, teaching courses and thereby proving your expert status than merely taking a melange of additional training.

One way to acquire new skills is to hire an assistant with approved training in the area. If the human factors in this relationship are compatible, he can teach you, on your own patients, the techniques you wish to acquire. If a long-term association is not part of your plan, he can be discarded as soon as you have the requisite skill and experience. Other patterns of exploitation are equally callous, depending upon the point of view. If someone is urging you to leave your training early to take advantage of some golden opportunity, remember that large organizations tend to consume people and talents as the most effective method of operation. They bring in the talent they need; and when it is obsolescent, they discard it for newer talent. If someone approaches you with inducements, expect to see adequate assurance in writing that you will be given the necessary educational leave to prevent your obsolescence as technology changes. Early obsolescence was not much of a factor in the past owing to the measured pace of medical progress, but the present frantic advances in the field have totally altered the rules of the game. Unless you can sidestep requirements by moving into purely administrative and management activities, you must keep up.

Consider the plight of the noninvasive cardiologist in a medium-size hospital. He may be helpless in the face of medical staff clamor for the services of an invasive cardiologist. The new man they want will bring to the hospital not only additional services and income but also prestige. But such a skill is not something one can pick up from reading. The only recourse of the department head, the noninvasive cardiologist, if he is to hold onto his position, is to personally recruit assistants with the skill. However, unless he is a very skillful negotiator, all he will have done is bring the competition into his own office.

One way to handle this problem, provided you are located reasonably near a medical school, is to have a teaching appointment in your specialty. As a formal instructor you will have the opportunity to become acquainted with the fellows and residents, assess their abilities both as human beings and as doctors, and perhaps pick an associate with whom you will be able to coexist and whose skills complement your own. Moreover, in your superior position as instructor, you can subtly steer away from your locale newcomers who might bring disastrous competition. Finally, a teaching position will not only satisfy some of your own continuing education requirements but will also serve to maintain your status as expert among your peers.

THE PRIVATE PRACTICE OPTION

For specialists with clinical skills who are considering the possibility of a private practice on the side, there are several important questions. The major one is this: Will you still be physically able to take the night and weekend calls when you are 55, 60, and 65? Your principal departmental activities may significantly influence your ability to operate efficiently during periods of high stress coupled with a demand for extra hours of clinical duties. The M.D. at 35 has a far greater physical capacity for coping with excessive demands than the same man at 60 or 70.

The issue is even more significant if you are a loner by nature and inclination. Unless you are certain you can control the level of clinical demand, you may be wiser to refrain from a career option in which output is directly related to your eroding physical stamina. You must assess your personal health prospects in terms of the data you possess about your own and your family's health history. If the position you are contemplating will allow you to descend gracefully (in terms of physical output) by relying, more and more, upon other people's skills, abilities, and stamina, then you are likely to have a very viable situation. But if you must continue delivering and if, when you fail, you will be replaced because of the paramount needs of the hospital and community, then perhaps another alternative would be advisable.

Another factor to consider in this same vein is the probably

personal effect arising from demographic changes in the population, particularly the quantity of chronic disease patients in your
field of expertise. Will the increase in demand for your services be
arithmetic or geometric? If the latter is more likely, can you assume
a clinical responsibility without realistic assurance of appropriate
logistic support from the institution? As previously discussed in
detail, getting help costs you on multiple levels. If you have already decided that is a price you do not wish to pay, then the
decision must influence your choice.

Of course, there is another common way to handle a rapidly
increasing demand: dilute the product. That may be a personally
feasible response to inordinate demands if you are entirely on your
own, but the situation changes when you have a hospital-based
position. As you divert increasing amounts of time from your departmental duties to satisfying patient demand, your satisfaction of
contractual obligations will drop and the chances of maintaining
your position will also. You never know, when you are cutting
corners, whether the corner cut is going to come back and haunt
you, particularly in light of the current emphasis on malpractice.

One way to maintain increasing output without significantly
reducing quality or paying the price of getting an assistant (competitor?) is to fully develop the nonprofessional assistant. There is
mounting pressure for specific physician assistants, a trend best
exemplified by the nurse anesthesist and the Fire/Rescue Paramedical Teams. The same augmentation of duties is occurring in many
of the newer, but as yet unregulated, hospital paramedical personnel. If you take that approach, you must realize both the immediate
hazards and the long-term consequences. The immediate costs are
your increased exposure and liability, potential reduction in income
(the fee for service varies with the qualifications of the delivering
agent), and the crisis that would result if this technician activity
were to suddenly stop because it was ruled illegal. The long-range
costs revolve around the use of such nonprofessional help by government and private corporations with a license to practice
medicine to control the activities of physicians more thoroughly.

SURVIVAL

Primitive society's simplistic and brutal method of deciding who is chief has been modified only partially in our present civilization. Although physical assault to unseat the leader is no longer employed, an assault on the leader's ego strength and credibility remains very much in use. In industry and business it is commonplace for the older man to be shoved aside abruptly by the younger challenger. Upon study, one observes that this occurs because the older leader allows himself the luxury of a self-delusion, which, while egotistically satisfying, becomes his Achilles heel. The fallacy is that he can do everything anyone else in his position can do. The moment the challenger can prove that he is, in fact, incapable of performing adequately, he is defeated by his own rules.

Perhaps in some situations the older leader can summarily remove challengers from the scene and maintain the fiction, but not conveniently in industry and even less so in medicine. With a growing number of talented people entering the field and striving for primacy, upsets in the leadership of hospital directorships may become common. The leader in the medical profession at least has the protection that, although not able to do everything, he has a wider experience than the challenger. If, however, he is so misguided as to think that his leadership depends upon the acquisition and adequate performance of all the latest medical techniques, it becomes relatively easy to beat him at his own power game. Although that may be a happy prospect for you when you are aspiring to the position of eminence, it may not be so attractive once you have arrived. So the director must make the point that his position depends upon his ability to manage people, and not upon his capacity to perform many specific techniques.

Your response to a challenge of leadership must include a survey of your constituency. Your position as leader depends upon the medical staff accepting you as a leader, and, as mentioned previously, you must anticipate ongoing changes in the composition of the medical staff that may subsequently alter the situation to one not in your favor. To best prepare yourself for the eventuality, you are advised to make a rapid survey of the age distribution of the medical staff, particularly those in power. If your acceptance as leader of the department is based to a large degree upon the support of physicians over the age of 55, you may expect to see that power base erode unless you are able to gain equal acceptance of the younger upcoming men. You may be certain that the younger men will be trained in a far different manner than your older colleagues were and will have greater and more precise expectations of the services that you are to provide. You must not only continue to satisfy the demands of the older power-wielders at the hospital but also be able to shift gears and satisfy the new physicians' demands for services.

Many people who rise swiftly to positions of eminence are intolerant of "anything second rate." By their definition, second rate is whatever they have not encountered before, whence the old folk saying "What is it? I don't like it!" The young gentlemen coming out of the centers of learning with their accent upon technology, often at the expense of a Gestalt approach, tend to play down the elements in their education that were not sufficiently impressed upon them and to play up those that were. So if you have developed pragmatic services that satisfy the needs of the medical staff but do not have the chrome-plated attractiveness of the university product, you may be in trouble. That is even more of a problem if you have trained in a relatively small institution without the full array of technology, talent, and models to play with. Thus it becomes important to determine if the rate at which the young are replacing the old exceeds the rate at which you can gradually accommodate to the new type of demand. That is, can you develop a following among the Young Turks?

No matter what your political connections in the circle of leadership, you can never be immune to the attacks of these Young Turks if their expectations are significantly undermet. Your attackers have one way of challenging you to which you have no reply. If they do not like what you are doing and you will not accommodate them, they can effectively counter any efforts you make simply by moving their area of clinical activity and their patients to another hospital. No one has enough political power to suffer that erosion of utilization and remain in the good graces of the top power echelon of the hospital. When your departmental activity drops, or fails to grow, you will be subject to harrassment from the top as well as from below, and that will further aggravate your problems of accommodation. So it is essential that you not underestimate the rising challenge of new men who could, depending upon the effort you put into public and hospital relations, become either your allies or your bitter enemies.

IMPACT OF INCOME CHANGES

Social change, for which there is tremendous potential in America today, may abruptly disrupt anyone's economic game plan. If one is prepared for change, he may avoid being forced into extreme positions or reactions. The changes may originate at various levels, as they have in California with the tremendous increase in premium for professional liability insurance. Those who were not prepared have been forced either to withdraw and seek non-insurance-required positions or to undertake other income-producing activities at the expense of their essential role in the hospital. As always, the abrupt responses with little forethought often have major short- and long-term costs.

Another change, one currently in an early stage of development, is the tendency for technology to spawn new departments that usually split off a portion of the action from an older department. The fortunate person in that new specialty suddenly has an important hospital base, but the director of the old department, with equal suddenness, finds his sphere of activity and consequently his income substantially decreased.

The greatest forays have occurred in the field of laboratory medicine, since from the beginning they provided virtually all the nonradiologic diagnostic services. A large number of subsidiary departments have subsequently split off from General Laboratory, and the process does not seem to have any reasonable end. In fact, very often you will find departments that have an array of diagnostic services far greater than that detailed under the Joint Commission. They are due entirely to the skill of a department manager in holding onto a coherent package of services and satisfying the majority interest and demand. As the new director your position is far less secure; you may take over a department only to find it suddenly reduced. So in effect, the attacks upon your security and activities may come from a multiplicity of directions.

The last attack upon your economic position may come from the increase in supply of specialists in your field. Presently, of course, most physicians choose their field for a variety of personal reasons that are unrelated to current job openings. There already is a considerable amount of planning at governmental levels with the ultimate aim of restricting the number of specialists in a field to the "apparent needs" of that field. The bureaucrats' plans may be good news for those who are in fields in which competition is keen, but those who have been in a buyer's market will regard the news differently. The paucity or surplus of young competitors will be of growing importance to you as you become more and more fixed in your own career path and as you enter the steeper portions of the ageing curve of decreasing abilities and reserve, when you will most need help.

THE NUMBER-TWO PROSPECTS

If you are in a field in which the supply of talent has been adequate for years, your only reasonable path to the directorship—unless you are prepared to move to some inaccessible area—is to begin at a lower spot on the ladder. This puts you on the other side of the coin discussed above, the side of the younger potential rival and adversary. Assuming that you have achieved the number-two spot, which may be difficult in a competitive field, what are your chances of obtaining the primary post? Will the chief retire soon enough that it is still reasonable for you to assume the mantle of leadership? As mentioned, doctors are a long-lived breed;

I know of some instances in which the prime assistant remained just that, the prime assistant. By the time the chief was ready to retire, the prime contender had become obsolete; and so a new man was brought in from the outside and the faithful servant never gained his just reward.

Obviously, to be in a number-two spot is a difficult, even a treacherous, arrangement unless you have some sort of definite agreement. If you affiliate with an older man in the expectation that, as he ages, he will step aside and allow a younger, more adequately trained man to take over, you may be making a very dangerous assumption. His very desire to get you as an assistant may be based upon his recognition of his failing abilities; if he can cozen you, he can live on your talents that produce his income. In the end you may become totally frustrated and worn out without ever realizing your full potential. As previously noted, institutions and powerful egos tend to consume other people for their own purposes.

If you are contemplating an assistant's position, it would be wise to have a frank talk about the projected career development open to you. What you require initially is to establish a firm association with the senior man; you need to be frank and appraise both his needs and yours. You need to reach a definite agreement to review the situation and your future in a year's time when the stability of the relationship has been established. At that time plan to work out some sort of formal agreement about sharing or transferring responsibility and its rewards. If rejected, you can always hope for erosion of time and ravages of disease to remove this stubborn man, but modern medicine may foil your hope. Otherwise, your only option is to begin the search anew.

CHARACTER ASSASSINATION

No matter what their training and career, humans make mistakes. Many mistakes are made early, and, depending upon the circumstances, they may be overlooked, accepted, or made much of. The problem, however, is not so much not making mistakes as it is avoiding their repetition. An obvious error even in this day of personal liberties and freedom is to offend a very influential person, one who takes the affront seriously and who makes sure that everyone knows just what a terrible person you are.

That type of whispering campaign is totally insidious; it cannot be directly countered except by (1) never letting it happen or, if it happens, (2) moving out of range. To stay and fight to regild your reputation is hopelessly idealistic. The more influential the person whom you have offended, the more extensive the spread of the mistruths, which can seriously constrict your options for years to come. A whispering campaign does not necessarily have to deal in facts. Indeed, it works much better if its basis in fact is minimal; for then it is elusive, insubstantial, and difficult to pin down. The black miasma of negative rumor travels much further than solid substantial fact.

There are innumerable cases of the young assistant who, by virtue of effectively doing a better than average job, has challenged and directly threatened his chief—and thereby demonstrated his political stupidity. If the young challenger does not back down, separation and pursuit by innuendo are inevitable. In all such instances, the lesser body is ejected from the greater one. Along with this separation, out goes the information about "he just wasn't the right man for that degree of responsibility." Those words, contrary to our experience with the evanescence of most words, have a half-life of years, not minutes or days, and they will continue to haunt the candidate for positions elsewhere for a very long time.

The author was recently consulted by a troubled hospital-based physician who felt that his career was in jeopardy, and he was entirely correct. Prior to receiving the request for the meeting, the author had already been told by several of his peers that the doctor was not the right man for his specialty. So this man's plea for advice and help was already tainted by the rumor that preceded him. Rumors such as that can ruin your career options in a local community because of the number of people who not only enjoy hearing the worst about someone but feel compelled to spread the "gospel" they have just heard. You need only look at the content of our media to confirm that, and note also the prominence given to corrections and retractions. So if you are a prickly, highly individualistic person, you must avoid running into an equally prickly, obstinate, and arrogant superior who will be glad to demonstrate his power over you by scuttling your career.

YOUR LIFESTYLE

Previously we have discussed your goals, strengths, ambitions, and work and the problems with work as related to your own personality. However, we have not specifically discussed your lifestyle, the one you have or the one you wish to develop. A most important question, first, is whether that lifestyle is compatible with your professional work. If it is not, your failure to recognize that crossroad fact may cause a mounting series of problems with ultimately disastrous consequences.

Obviously, your lifestyle is not merely your own; it is an amalgam of the hopes, dreams, and desires of your wife and your children as well. Since so much of it is unconscious or below the limits of your awareness, you may not be able to easily vocalize and examine it. All too often you seize upon a single static objective as if it were the essence of your M.O. But such an objective as "I am to retire at 65 with a net worth of half a million" is a closed-end type of plan that fails to take into account any of the innumerable changes that take place on your way to 65.

What you and your wife need is an open-ended plan that will enable you to adapt to changing circumstances and opportunities. The very fact that you purchase life, sickness, and disability insurance acknowledges your appreciation of the complete variability of life events. People readily lump together many goals in a single generalized statement such as living in Suburb X and retiring in Y Town. In analyzing their patterns of living, however, you will find that they actually subscribe to a multiple series of goals rather than a single set. However, those goals often occur in a certain preestablished order that must be maintained to generate the life satisfaction that is the ultimate broad objective.

To give a single example, if you undertake a practice option that requires being available on frequent calls and emergencies, then you must live reasonably close to the locus of such activity. Your family, however, may have their hearts set upon living in an area far more attractive and far more distant. There are obviously a varying number of compromises possible in such a situation; but if the solution chosen veers to either extreme, it will lead to a downstream change in the family relationship or in your work or both, none of which was planned for or desired.

Most busy physicians respond to decreased family contact by attempting to substitute dollars for minutes spent, but the substitution is not a viable alternative. While children are young, you are somehow able to fit them into the nooks and crannies of your irregular hours of leisure. However, when school schedules appear, there is little flexibility on either side, and your areas of mutual contact may shrink to an unacceptable minimum. Thus further conflict is generated, since your free time and that of the family may become totally out of phase.

The point is not that you should avoid parenthood—to avoid such crises—but that decisions made now have consequences that can logically be worked out. Otherwise, you may gradually become so busy satisfying demand and generating income that you may lose sight of the purpose of your existence. Your family may be unable to recognize the dilemma you are in, a dilemma due in part to your misinterpretation of their desires, and may thus aggravate rather than help.

We are all living examples of Parkinson's law, namely, that work or activity expands to fill the time available for it. As we get older and as we see more need for our efforts, we tend to get busier. When younger, we tend to ignore events that, because of lack of appropriate background, seem to be of little or no consequence. But ten or fifteen years later we recognize the implications in those events and thus devote attention and time. Thus as you age and mature, if you are politically astute, you will move into the councils of power and will find that, as a consequence, you will have to take more time, not less, to accomplish tasks. To change the course of action with brains rather than brawn takes more time planning and executing than does a Kamikaze frontal attack. As you develop a more complex operation and its complex problems, you must spend more time developing and cultivating additional contacts.

One of the key factors you must examine at reasonably frequent intervals is the amount, nature, and volume of nonessential activities that are recurrent. As you get busier and more involved, there are a myriad of little extra things to be done. Some you must personally take care of, but cannot the balance be delegated to someone else? If you are forced to do far more driving on a regular basis than you had ever planned, consider the time and the cost. At a certain point it would be more practical to pay someone so you can properly concentrate upon your profession. As a manager you have to take upon yourself the task of managing even your own activities more efficiently. Certainly anyone who reads about the aristocrats and the very rich notices that they have subcontracted every nonessential activity so they can concentrate upon their main tasks. Physicians, while not extremely rich, are a well-paid group in terms of hourly earnings. It would seem logical, therefore, to delegate every minor but essential time-wasting task to someone at a lower hourly rate.

MOTIVATION

According to current theory, humanity strives initially for security, self-preservation, food, and shelter, all of which the American doctor has in plentitude. Following satisfaction of those basic needs, humans seek group acceptance and social status; again the doctor is well provided for. A more sophisticated motivational force is independence, and the license to practice medicine liberally bestows that upon the physician. The freedom and ability to change career direction is even further removed from basic need, yet for the physician that may, at his level, be basic.

It is likely you will want to continue doing different things at different stages of your life with respect to both work and lifestyle.

Certainly facing all of us is the most radical change, the transition from active work to a state of retirement. Normally the transition will occur only when the physician is financially prepared for it, so that the drive of financial solvency is muted; he can shift gears easily to a lower level of work. Of course, illness and disablement may cause a radical change in work and career direction, but even so the physician has more resources than others in his community. The smoothness of the transitional phase depends upon the amount of extrinsic pressures leveled at the physician: the degree of planning and forethought invested and the resources accumulated in anticipation of such need.

THE IDENTITY CRISIS

Even if your department grows at a minimal rate of 10 percent per year, in eight-plus years the activity will have doubled. Activities of management that originally occupied only a small percentage of your time will double and then triple if you are consistently successful. Management may now occupy most of your time. As doctors, we have all been programmed to feel that our main business is doctoring, and only the diagnostic and nonclinical specialists need no such reassurance.

Thus the older hospital-based physician may suffer a crisis of uncertainty about his worth when he suddenly realizes that he no longer is providing "real patient care services." Since most physicians are social creatures working with people and alongside compatriots, the most innocent jibes of these selfsame peers may be the trigger that sets off an identity crisis. That happens most often in institutions with well-organized hierarchial structures in which, as you climb the ladder of success, you gradually move further and further away from doctoring. At some point in time the physician may suddenly decide to chuck it all and go out and become a real doctor again. Whether that is an attempt to recapture his independence or his youth or again feed his ego or whatever, it is a common enough occurrence to warrant mention.

If the medical director keeps a close check on his career course, he will be aware of the gradual shift from a mix of clinical and managerial to a purely administrative phase. If the tendency is undesirable, he can easily correct it by delegating paperwork rather than patient care. Attempting a major course correction, without planning, late in your career may be unwise for a variety of reasons. The most pertinent reason is that, if you have not actually been utilizing and practicing those skills for years, your patient care efforts will be inadequate no matter how great your desire. You will have abandoned a secure and stable, albeit dull, course in which you have been providing useful services for a new endeavor in which you are not properly suited.

THE JOKER

In all of your long-range career planning you must be aware of the joker factor. All humans are prey to trauma, illness, and imbalance that can suddenly take someone out of action and thereby change the entire game. That is more apt to happen to the more senior members of the hospital's staff structure. Thus a particularly favored position with a senior solon could be an unreliable keystone in your career arch. There are any number of health and personal factors that can render a man less effective, particularly in times of stress. Radical changes may appreciably alter the priorities you have assigned to various goals.

CLOSING OUT

Do you plan to work until something makes you no longer able to work and only then prepare for retirement? Or have you a proposed schedule for phasing out? Obviously, the closer you get to 65 the more detailed and precise your answers should be. As mentioned previously, you have planned your medical career and that of your specialization and you have conducted a department over the years, so you have had training in rational and reasonable short- and long-term planning. Thus there is no excuse for you not to have addressed yourself similarly to the terminal portions of your career. That is of particular importance if you have been toying with the idea of a midcourse career correction or a late career change. Unless you keep up your feedback from all the persons involved in your future, you may find that whatever plans you had are unrealistic; instead of gradually phasing out, you may find yourself suddenly dropped at a time not personally auspicious.

As a professional you must continue to give as much thought to the institution employing you as to your own plans, since the institution expects to continue in existence long after you are gone. At some point your value to it may be so minimal that, no matter what your political strength, you will have to step aside. In business, that is commonly known as being kicked upstairs. You may find yourself director emeritus in charge of nothing because your assistant director is now handling the whole show. You will also find that the emeritus status has a significant negative influence on your income, unless you have a cast-iron contract.

This is not the time to go into full-time patient care to earn your living, especially not with the "I'll show them" attitude. If instead you have been approaching this late career period by looking for low-demand, low-income options, you may really be ready for quasi retirement. Provided positions that are suitable to your talents are available, this may be a reasonable method of phasing out. Depending upon the community you are in, the institution, and your individual circumstances, you may have a lot of help and opportunity in making the transition or none at all.

Directors of departments with no clinical responsibility, such as laboratory and x-ray, are in a uniquely advantageous position at this time. They can easily, if they choose, begin shifting the major burden of activities upon their younger associates or partners and continue to provide some services for which they can receive income for a number of years. That, of course, is contingent upon whether or not they are professionally competent to perform those services.

But if you have clinical responsibilities that you know you cannot adequately satisfy because of your increasing physical limitations, what is your alternative? If you have the financial resources, you may retire. Otherwise, you must consider some other transition to final retirement. A reasonable alternative is to seek a staff position with some institution, but that requires a considerable amount of forethought and planning. You must remember that most institutions will not hire a man who is at or near the mandatory retirement age. Therefore, if you wish to make the transition to a less demanding, more economically stable position, you must do so while your value to the new organization is still reasonably great. That means you should be preparing to look for an alternative position while you are in your mid-fifties rather than your mid-sixties.

The best way to get a perspective on retirement is to talk to the physicians at your institution who have retired or who are on the verge of retiring. Certainly their immediate practical experience will help make you aware of problems that cannot be anticipated and of just what measures of planning will be required. As with any other form of gentle cross-examination, the quizzing should take place in a social setting with the use of some libation to loosen the tongue.

MANDATORY RETIREMENT

It may be that you are so politically potent at the hospital that no one dares retire you until you drop or die. However, old doctors are human and so suffer from the infirmities of age. Your absence for recurrent illness and slow recuperation may be cumulatively greater than you had anticipated, and greater too than the institution can tolerate. In that case it is unlikely that you can hold onto the prime position to the very end. Perhaps at one time you were number two and had a chief who literally had to be carried out of the department and placed in a nursing home before you could take over the position. If so, you should ask yourself whether the same thing can happen again. Humans characteristically have a blind spot for their own inadequacies: "It can't happen to me because I'm different." However, when you are 68 or 72, they may also have to carry you out of the hospital and put you in a nursing home. At that point the struggle to maintain your position will merely accentuate any problems you may have had.

Many retiring physicians go into the business of managing their own estates, their money, and their investments. That is much like asking a medical student to do brain surgery. Unless you have thoroughly trained yourself in business affairs during the last decade of your career, you had best leave those affairs in the hands of the persons who have been handling them up to now. Limit your contribution to kibitzing and advice on a more frequent basis. Otherwise, you are apt to reduce your financial reserves to the point at which retirement is a financial burden and not a pleasure.

FAMILY PLANS

If you expect to still be married by the time of your retirement, you must give attention to your spouse's needs and plans. If the children are her prime preoccupation, there may be little need to worry about her other goals. But once the kids have grown and gone, you and she must direct attention to her own plans for closing out. Unless you coordinate your plans, you may be heading east while she is going west.

You may both wish to live somewhere else during retirement but have trouble agreeing upon where that somewhere else is. One of your considerations must be whether any given locale is actually reasonable for you. Moving after you have retired is often very unwise because you have left yourself little time for preparations and emergencies. If you plan to move to a place reasonably accessible to your present residence, you ought to investigate the area well in advance so that you can make some initial commitment and investment. That not only provides a base to begin visiting on your holidays and vacations but also builds up a second area of personal connections and familiarities to ease the tremendous dislocation that can come with total cessation of "useful activity."

Certainly in the last quarter of your life you may need more help from others than you have ever needed before. It may be possible for you to purchase most of that help if you are well set up financially. Otherwise, you may have to depend upon the goodwill of others, and it is difficult to generate such goodwill in large amounts on short notice.

TERMINAL SPECIALIZATION

You know from following patients that the rate of loss of function is quite variable and is dependent upon a myriad of individual factors. Similarly, as you yourself age, some functions will persist at a useful level while others deteriorate or fail altogether. Thus as you grow older you must also grow more insightful. You must be aware of what you can still do well and what you cannot do at all. Obviously, one thing you can do increasingly well is look at any problem with far greater wisdom and experience than a younger person.

Whether you have kept your technical expertise up to a useful level may be another matter. Many physicians talk about going into teaching when they retire. In general, however, that is wishful thinking, since most physicians expect to go out and teach what they themselves learned twenty or more years ago. Also, at an advanced age, their resilience to challenge and change may be far less than is required by the interaction between student and teacher. In fact, if you observe carefully, most emeritus professors no longer have regular classes because they can't stand those insufferable snips who behave so disgracefully.

So unless you have some special, needed attribute, you had best settle upon some second career other than teaching. The location you choose for retirement activity may have as much influence upon your opportunities as any individual skills you may possess. Thus you may easily decide your second career option negatively by giving inadequate thought to the site of your retirement residence. Of course, when you are 40 years old, 65 seems very distant, but the choices you make at 40 may drastically amplify or restrict the options available to you 20 years later. All of us have seen physicians who could not let go until they were shut out of their activities by their very incompetence. That is a dreadful way to conclude a productive career. Those physicians have had people dependent on them for decades; but when their very incompetence drives away their patients, the patients, on leaving, remember them for their current mistakes rather than for their past glories. We should take a lesson from that and prepare to leave earlier and more gracefully.

APPENDIX A

GUIDELINES CONCERNING THE PROVISIONS IN THE RADIOLOGIST-HOSPITAL CONTRACT*

INTRODUCTION

The purpose of these guidelines is to assist radiologists and hospitals in negotiating or revising contracts to meet the requirements of California law and to aid in maintaining existing mutually satisfactory relationships.

The radiological department in a hospital exists for the benefit of sick and injured persons; and in that hospital most of the responsibility for radiologic examinations and treatments rests on radiologists who practice there. A department of radiology, like any other basic unit of a hospital, must have a chief in order to function in the best interests of patients, referring physicians, the hospital itself and the community. The chief of the radiological department should be medically responsible to the medical staff and administratively responsible to the Board of Trustees through the administration.

GUIDELINE I: *Selection and Medical Staff Appointment*
    A. Selection of the radiologist in a hospital and his appoint-

* Board of Medical Examiners, Department of Consumer Affairs, State of California, 1020 N Street, Sacramento, Calif. 95814.

ment to the medical staff of the hospital is the concern of both the medical staff and the governing board of that hospital.

B. The medical staff shall have the right to recommend appointment to or removal from the staff of a radiologist in a hospital, but the ultimate responsibility for decision rests with the governing board of the hospital.

C. The type of contractual relationship between the radiologist and the hospital should be acceptable to the Executive Committee of the medical staff.

The California State Board of Medical Examiners has announced that the contractual relationship created between the physician and the hospital must not only be in accordance with the approved guidelines, but also in compliance with the Medical Practice Act including, where applicable, Business and Professions Code sections 650 (unearned rebates, refunds and discounts) and 2392.5 (prohibiting fee splitting).

GUIDELINE II: *Independent Contractor*

The contract should state and assure that the radiologist is an independent contractor.

> COMMENT: It should be understood and agreed that the radiologist is at all times acting and performing as an independent contractor practicing his profession of medicine and specializing in radiology for the benefit of the patient. This fact notwithstanding, the radiologist has a responsibility to the governing board of the hospital to conduct his practice with competence and thoroughness so that it and the facility also protect the interests of the institution. All applicable provisions of law relating to licensing and regulating of physicians and hospitals shall be fully complied with by both parties.

GUIDELINE III: *Termination Clause*

The contract may provide that it may be terminated by either party upon written notice of a given period of time. When the hospital desires to terminate the contract, then the Executive Committee of the medical staff shall be consulted by the administration.

GUIDELINE IV: *Medical Staff Membership and Privileges*

A. Prior to practicing in a hospital, a radiologist shall apply, and be accepted, as a member of the hospital staff in accordance with the medical staff's by-laws, and in the same manner as other physicians.

B. With the same consideration as any other member of ·the medical staff, the radiologist shall be extended or denied privileges in the hospital, including the privilege of admitting patients into the hospital for the purposes of performing complex diagnostic procedures and/or treatment.

GUIDELINE V: *Professional Liability Insurance*

A. The radiologist is to be treated essentially in the same manner as other members of the medical staff concerning professional liability insurance.

B. The contract may specify the requirements and limits of professional liability coverage.

> COMMENT: Even though a hospital-based physician is not an employee of the hospital, the hospital may still be liable for his malpractice on a theory of ostensible authority. *Seneris v. Haas,* 45 C.2d 811, 291 P.2d 915. (1955).

> *Rosner v. Peninsula Hospital District,* 224 Cal.App.2d 115, 36 Cal.Rptr. 332 (1964) holds that the Board of district hospitals, because of special limitations in the district hospital law, cannot deny medical staff membership on the sole ground that the physician does not have malpractice insurance. Subparagraph B is designed to give the district hospital protection for the acts of the hospital-based physician.

GUIDELINE VI: *Department Rules and Regulations*

Policies relating to the standards of professional practice and the duties of the radiologist are primarily the concerns of the medical staff, and they shall be described in the medical staff and radiological department rules and regulations instead of the hospital-radiologist contract. The operating policies should be consistent with the general policies of the hospital. In the event of disagreement, the matter may be referred to the Executive Committee of the medical staff supplemented by a radiologist.

> COMMENT: The radiologist should have definite and adequate hours of attendance in the department to permit ample time for performance and consultation in every examination and treatment.

He should participate in the educational and committee activities of the medical staff.

GUIDELINE VII: *Selection of Equipment*

The radiologist who is to be Chairman of the department shall advise and participate with the hospital in the selection of equipment and the provisions for its maintenance. He should annually project department space, personnel and equipment needs for the calendar year and tentative projected needs for the coming years. He shall be responsible for the establishment of standards for the control of radiation hazards and the general administration of the department.

GUIDELINE VIII: *Personnel*

The selection and retention of technicians, nurses, secretaries and other nonprofessional personnel in the department shall be subject to the approval of the hospital and the radiologist. Personnel policies for vacation time, sick leave, etc., shall be consistent with the personnel policies for other hospital personnel.

COMMENT: This guideline leaves options for the radiologist to assume various degrees of responsibility in personnel management.

GUIDELINE IX: *Professional Compensation*

Fee for service agreements and contracts based on the sharing of reasonable and equitable percentages of gross charges are acceptable methods of compensation. Lease arrangements based on reasonable charges for the rental of space and/or equipment are also acceptable. Contracts based on a percentage of net income are not acceptable. Other forms of contracts must be individually evaluated to determine whether or not they are acceptable.

The California State Board of Medical Examiners has announced that contracts based on a sharing of reasonable and equitable percentages of gross charges are an acceptable method of compensation provided the portion of the fees received by the hospital is commensurate with the expenses, direct or indirect, incurred by the hospital in connection with the furnishings or the facilities.

COMMENT: Fee for Service Contracts.

A fee for service contract would allow for the specific dollar amount that a radiologist is to collect for each examination. This type of contract would separate and define for the patient charges which represent the hospital costs and charges which represent the radiologist's professional fees.

COMMENT: Percentage of Gross Contracts.

The allocation of a percentage of gross charges is a financial arrangement for dividing gross income between radiologists and hospitals. Under such an arrangement, the radiologist pays the hospital, or receives from the hospital, a percentage of gross billings.

A majority of the contracts in California and the United States are percentage of gross contracts. The percentage of gross contract has been held to be legal in *Blank v. Palo Alto Stanford Medical Center*, 234 Cal.App.2d 377 (1965) and *Letsch v. Northern San Diego County Hospital District*, 246 Cal.App.2d 673 (1966), where that portion of the fees received by the hospital was commensurate with the expenses, direct and indirect, incurred by the hospital in connection with the furnishings or the facilities.

COMMENT: Lease Arrangements.

The lease usually includes the services and utilities such as heat, light, water, elevator, janitor. building repair and maintenance, and similar services. The equipment may or may not be included, but the radiologist usually provides the necessary supplies and personnel. The rental should be based on a charge per unit of space and/or equipment and it should include a reasonable return on the hospital's investment. The charge should not be based on a percentage of gross revenue.

GUIDELINE X: *Responsibility for Costs*

The contract between the hospital and the radiologist should state the costs that are to be borne by the hospital and those that are to be borne by the radiologist.

GUIDELINE XI: *Billing*

When there is a fee for service contract, the radiologist's professional fee and the hospital's charge should be billed separately or separately itemized on the patient's bill. When there is a total charge which includes professional fees, this fact and the name(s) of the radiologist(s) should be made known to the patient.

GUIDELINE XII: *Charges*

Schedules for radiologist's professional fees and the hospital's charges may be prepared by the radiologist and the hospital independently or together. Each should be informed of the other's charges. Professional fees should be in accordance with local customary fees for comparable services. If there is a disagreement about such charges or proposed changes in charges, the matter should be referred to existing medical peer review organizations or to the Executive Committee of the medical staff of the hospital.

APPENDIX B

GUIDELINES CONCERNING THE PROVISIONS IN THE PATHOLOGIST-HOSPITAL CONTRACT*

INTRODUCTION

These guidelines are prepared to aid pathologists and hospitals in negotiating or revising contracts to meet the requirements of California law. The goal is not to define an ideal type of arrangement, but to eliminate illegal arrangements. These guidelines are designed to recognize the combined role of the pathologist as a physician and department administrator responsible to the medical staff for those duties which are the primary concern of the medical staff. It is hoped that they are sufficiently broad and flexible to enable pathologists and hospitals to retain their mutually satisfactory arrangements.

The California State Board of Medical Examiners has announced that in reviewing the contracts it will also consider that the contractual relationship created between the physician and the hospital must not only be in accordance with the approved guidelines but also in compliance with the Medical Practice Act, including, where applicable, Business and Professions Code sec-

*Board of Medical Examiners, Department of Consumer Affairs, State of California, 1020 N Street, Sacramento, Calif. 95814.

255

tions 650 (unearned rebates, refunds and discounts) and 2392.5 (prohibiting fee splitting).

GUIDELINE I

The pathologist is to be a member of the active medical staff of the hospital and a member of the Department of Pathology. One pathologist shall be chairman of the Department of Pathology.

GUIDELINE II

A. The pathologist is to be treated in essentially the same manner as other members of the medical staff concerning malpractice insurance.

B. The contract may specify the requirements and limits of malpractice coverage.

> COMMENT: Even though a hospital-based physician is not an employee of the hospital, the hospital may still be liable for his malpractice on a theory of ostensible authority. *Seneris v. Haas*, 45 C.2d 811, 291 P.2d 915 (1955).
>
> *Rosner v. Peninsula Hospital District*, 224 Cal.App.2d 115, 36 Cal.Rptr. 332 (1964) holds that the Boards of district hospitals, because of special limitations in the district hospital law, cannot deny medical staff membership on the sole ground that the physician does not have malpractice insurance. Subparagraph B is designed to give the district hospital protection for the acts of hospital-based physicians.

GUIDELINE III

The pathologist should be responsible for recommendations concerning the acquisition of laboratory equipment.

> COMMENT: Assessment of the need for new equipment and the selection of specific items to fill that need should be based on evaluations and justifications made by the staff pathologist.

GUIDELINE IV

The selection and retention of laboratory personnel shall be subject to the approval of the pathologist and the hospital. Laboratory personnel policies should be consistent with the personnel policies for other hospital departments.

> COMMENT: This guideline leaves options for the pathologist to assume various degrees of responsibility in personnel management.

GUIDELINE V

The standards of medical practice and duties of the pathologist are primarily the concerns of the medical staff. Such standards are to be described in the department rules and regulations of the medical staff rather than be included in the hospital-pathologist contract.

> COMMENT: Examples of such clauses include:
> A. Consultation services of the pathologist.
> B. Participation in educational activities.
> C. Medical staff activities.
> In the event of a disagreement between the pathologist and the hospital as to the quality of care, the matter shall be referred to the Executive Committee of the Medical Staff.

GUIDELINE VI

Fee for service is an acceptable form of billing practice. Compensation to the pathologist may take the form of a separately billed or separately itemized professional fee or a reasonable and equitable percentage of gross revenue. These are not the only acceptable types of contracts.

The California State Board of Medical Examiners has announced that the contracts based on a sharing of reasonable and equitable percentages of gross charges are an acceptable method of compensation provided the portion of the fees received by the hospital is commensurate with the expenses, direct or indirect, incurred by the hospital in connection with the furnishings or the facilities.

The percentage of net revenue contracts are not acceptable.

Lease arrangements together with services by lessor may be acceptable if the amount of rent paid is reasonable for the amount and type of space and services leased.

> COMMENT: Percentage of Gross Contracts.
> A majority of contracts in California and the United States are percentage of gross contracts. The percentage of gross contract has been held to be legal in *Blank v. Palo Alto Stanford Medical Center*, 234 Cal.App.2d 377 (1965) and *Letsch v. Northern San Diego County Hospital District*, 246 Cal.App. 2d 673 (1966), where that portion of the fees received by the hospital was commensurate with the expenses, direct and indirect, incurred by the hospital in connection with the furnishings of the facilities.

> COMMENT: Separately Itemized or Separately Billed Professional
>   Fee Contracts.
> A. This type of contract sets the specific dollar amount that a pathologist is to collect for each test. It separates and defines labo-

ratory charges which represent the hospital overhead from those charges which represent the professional and administrative fees of the pathologist.

B. This maintains the current and mutually satisfactory compensation to each party. These guidelines are not intended to modify the present income level of the pathologist or the hospital.

GUIDELINE VII

The contract between the hospital and pathologist should state the costs that are to be borne by the hospital and those that are to be borne by the pathologist.

COMMENT: Examples of costs are: Salaries of technical personnel, clinical personnel, equipment, supplies, telephone, utilities and other supportive services.

GUIDELINE VIII

If the laboratory charge includes the professional fees of the pathologist, this fact should be made known to the patient.

COMMENT: This guideline may be fulfilled in a number of different ways. The pathologist who bills separately is already identified to the patient. When combined billing procedures are used, the bill may list the professional component for each charge or may contain a statement that this component is included in the present charge.

GUIDELINE IX

Independent Contractor. The contract should state and assure that the pathologist is an independent contractor.

COMMENT: It should be understood and agreed that the pathologist is at all times acting and performing as an independent contractor practicing his profession of medicine and surgery and specializing in pathology. All applicable provisions of law relating to licensing and regulating of physicians and hospitals should be fully complied with by both parties.

GUIDELINE X

Termination Clause. The contract may provide that it may be terminated by either party upon written notice of a given period of time. The executive committee of the medical staff shall be consulted before any such action is taken.

COMMENT: As a member of the medical staff, the pathologist is to be extended or denied privileges in the hospital with the same consideration as any other member.

GUIDELINE XI

The pathologist's professional fees should be in general accordance with customary local fees for comparable services.

The schedule of total charges for laboratory procedures should be prepared by the pathologist and hospital. If there is disagreement about such charges or proposed changes in such charges, the matter should be referred to the Executive Committee of the Medical Staff or to a local medical peer review organization.

REFERENCES

1. A. R. Lamb, *The Presbyterian Hospital and the Columbia-Presbyterian Medical Center, 1868-1943* (New York: Columbia University Press, 1955).

2. R. L. Yanda, *The Management of Respiratory Care Services* (New York: Projects in Health, Inc., 1976).

3. *Accreditation Manual for Hospitals* (Chicago: Joint Commission on Accreditation of Hospitals, 1970, updated 1973).

4. R. L. Yanda, op. cit.

5. M. R. Haig and M. B. Sussman, "Professionalization and Unionism," *American Behavioral Scientist*, Vol. 14 (1971), pp. 525-540.

6. A. C. Filley and R. J. House, *Managerial Process and Organizational Behavior* (Glenview, Ill.: Scott, Foresman & Company, 1969).

7. S. Levey and N. P. Loomba, *Health Care Administration* (Philadelphia: J. B. Lippincott Co., 1973).

8. H. B. Pickle, *Personality and Success*, Small Business Administration Research Series No. 4 (Washington, D.C.: GOP, 1964).

9. J. R. Payne, T. J. Braunstein, J. M. Ketchel, and M. C. Pease, *A Brief Survey of Potential Decision Aids*, NTIS Study AD-AO-16627 (Washington, D.C.: Office of Naval Research, 1975), p. 17.

10. D. McGregor, *Leadership and Motivation* (Cambridge, Mass.: The M.I.T. Press, 1966).

11. A. H. Maslow, "A Theory of Human Motivation," in R. J. Lowry (Ed.), *Self-Esteem, Self-Actualization: Germinal Papers of A. H. Maslow* (Monterey, Calif.: Brooks/Cole Publ., 1973).

12. L. L. Weed, *Medical Records, Medical Education and Patient Care* (Cleveland: Case Western Reserve University Press, Yearbook Distrib., 1969).

13. D. B. Starkweather, "The Rationale for Decentralization in Large Hospitals," *Hospital Administration*, Vol. 15 (Spring 1970), pp. 27-45.

14. R. Schulz and A. C. Johnson, "Conflict in Hospitals," *Hospital Administration*, Vol. 16 (Spring 1971), pp. 36–50.

15. V. C. Medvei, "Teams and Their Leaders," *Lancet*, Vol. i (1964).
16. L. W. Porter, E. E. Lawler III, and J. R. Hackman, *Behavior in Organizations* (New York: McGraw-Hill Book Company, 1975), p. 428.
17. Ibid., pp. 429, 431, 432.
18. P. Pigors and C. A. Meyers, *Personnel Administration*, 7th Ed. (New York: McGraw-Hill Book Company, 1975), Chap. 9.
19. J. B. Miner, *The Management Process: Theory, Research and Practice* (New York: The Macmillan Company, 1973), p. 267.
20. P. R. Lawrence, "How to Deal with Resistance to Change," *Harvard Business Review*, Vol. 32 (1954), p. 56.
21. M. Smith, "Functioning as a Professional, Not as a Technician," in "Definition of Quality Care," *Annals of the Royal College of Physicians & Surgeons of Canada*, Vol. 7 (October 1974), No. 4, pp. 289-290.
22. V. C. Medvei, op. cit.
23. L. W. Porter et al., op. cit., pp. 457, 458.
24. R. C. Sampson, *How to Survive the Business Rat Race* (New York: McGraw-Hill Book Company, 1970), pp. 184-186.
25. B. J. Speroff, "The Identification of Informal Leaders," *Hospital Administration*, Vol. 10 (Spring 1965), pp. 42-52.
26. E. B. Flippo, *Principles of Personnel Management* (New York: McGraw-Hill Book Company, 1976), p. 444.
27. M. J. Gannon, "The Management of Peripheral Employees," *Personnel Journal*, Vol. 54 (1975), No. 9, p. 482.
28. T. K. Oh, "Human Motivation in Management Theory—History and Trends," *Industrial Management*, 14:10 (October 1972).
29. F. Luthans, *Introduction to Management: A Contingency Approach* (New York: McGraw-Hill Book Company, 1976).
30. J. N. Pfifner and R. P. Sherwood, *Administrative Organization* (Englewood Cliffs, N.J.: Prentice-Hall, Inc., 1960), pp. 56, 57.
31. F. Luthans, op. cit.
32. J. L. Massie and J. Douglas, *Managing: A Contemporary Introduction* (Englewood Cliffs, N.J.: Prentice-Hall, Inc., 1973).
33. C. Argyris, "Human Problems with Budgets," *Harvard Business Review*, January–February 1953.
34. E. Dale, *Management: Theory and Practice*, 3rd Ed. (New York: McGraw-Hill Book Company, 1973).
35. J. H. Knowles, "The Hospital," *Scientific American*, Vol. 293 (1973), No. 3, pp. 128-137.
36. *Accreditation Manual for Hospitals*, op. cit.
37. S. J. Miller, *Prescription for Leadership* (Chicago: Aldine Press, 1970).
38. J. Ludwig, "A Letter to the Next Speaker," *Mayo Clinic Proceedings*, 40:807 (1973).

INDEX